Business Strategies for a Caring Profession

A PRACTITIONER'S GUIDEBOOK

Sharon L. Yenney, CBY Associates

American Psychological Association Practice Directorate

AMERICAN PSYCHOLOGICAL ASSOCIATION, WASHINGTON, DC

A Cautionary Note:

This manual was written to serve both as a reference and as a tool to help psychologists practice more effectively and efficiently in a changing, demanding marketplace. The information contained herein is accurate and complete to the best of our knowledge. However, *Business Strategies for a Caring Profession: A Practitioner's Guidebook* should be read with the understanding that it is meant as a supplement, not a substitute, for sound legal, accounting, business, or other professional consulting services. When such services are required, the assistance of a competent professional should be sought.

Published by
American Psychological Association
750 First Street, NE
Washington, DC 20002

Copies may be ordered from
APA Order Department
P.O. Box 2710
Hyattsville, MD 20784

Typeset in Century by Easton Publishing Services, Inc., Easton, MD

Printer: Kirby Lithographic Company, Inc., Arlington, VA
Cover designer: Berg Design, Albany, NY
Technical/production editor: Susan Bedford

Library of Congress Cataloging-in-Publication Data

Yenney, Sharon.
    Business strategies for a caring profession : a practitioner's guidebook / Sharon L. Yenney & American Psychological Association Practice Directorate.
        p.   cm.
    Includes bibliographical references.
    ISBN 1-55798-254-6
    1. Clinical psychology—Practice—United States.   I. CBY Associates.   II. American Psychological Association. Practice Directorate.   III. Title.
    RC467.95.Y46   1994
    616.89′0068—dc20
                                                    94-13771
                                                    CIP

Printed in the United States of America
First Edition

Contents

Forms, Charts, and Worksheets

See page 119 for a listing of Practice Analysis Tools included in the Appendix.

Foreword

Few mental health professionals acquire the business skills necessary to succeed in today's market from their clinical training. Rapid change in the marketplace has made it even more difficult to quickly adjust to change. Yet, psychologists are uniquely trained and are well situated to take advantage of the tremendous opportunities in today's market.

As the market shifts toward organized and integrated systems of care, your response will require planning and hard work. As Peter Drucker once stated, "Future success will not just happen if one works hard enough. It requires decisions—now. It imposes risk—now. It demands allocation of resources, and above all, of human resources—now. It requires work—now."

The Practice Directorate is strongly committed to providing our members with information, guidance, and leadership. Despite this Guidebook's focus on the business of providing psychological care, we do not mean to indicate that maintaining high clinical standards is secondary. We believe that both the clinical and business sides of a psychological practice are important for a successful future.

Acknowledgments

We are grateful for the contributions of the following people whose hard work and assistance have made this book possible: Sharon L. Yenney, Russ Newman, PhD, JD, Henry Engleka, Dan Abrahamson, PhD, Rick Reckman, PhD, George Taylor, PhD, Anita Brown, PhD, Mike Sullivan, PhD, Shirley Higuchi, JD, and Paul Herndon, as well as the APA Practice Directorate Marketing Department staff including Neela Agarwalla, JD, Garth Huston, Brian Schilling, and Chris Vein.

1

Introduction

The Need for a Guidebook

The United States is witnessing a dramatic alteration in the manner in which health and mental health services are funded, organized, and delivered. Vigorous efforts by large and small purchasers of health and mental health services to reduce costs have placed more and more demands on practicing psychologists. From the intrusion of third parties into the client–therapist relationship to demands of financial risk sharing arrangements, practitioners are being forced to seek new answers to questions concerning the most effective and sustainable method of delivering services.

For all who feel the force of these winds of change, this Guidebook was created to put the changes in perspective and to offer guidance for maintaining a viable, profitable practice. Most practitioners are experiencing the impact of this movement to "corporatize" American health care. Surviving the changes will require using your clinical training in new and innovative ways.

This Guidebook is also a response to the practicing psychologists who have called or written the American Psychological Association (APA) Practice Directorate for assistance in solving business questions related to their practices. From these questions, it became clear that a comprehensive, organized approach to the business operations of psychological practices was needed. This Guidebook is a place to turn for guidance about the business of operating a psychological practice.

Finally, it is clear that the once distinct fields of physical and mental health care overlap considerably. More and more, the services provided by psychologists reflect their integration into the larger health care community. In recognition of this, we have used the terms *mental health services* and *health services* interchangeably throughout the guidebook.

Goals of the Guidebook

The goals of this Guidebook are twofold. The primary purpose is to provide information that will help psychologists select an appropriate model for practice, establish the business policies and procedures that will make each practice effective and efficient, and position it to compete in the marketplace. The second purpose is to motivate practitioners to assess their business operations on a regular basis so that they remain viable in a changing and challenging health care environment.

As you read through this manual, keep in mind that it will *not* attempt to provide you with a detailed, fail-proof, step-by-step plan for making your practice more effective and profitable; such a plan is simply impossible. One reason is that an effective, thriving practice in northern California may look very different from a similarly prosperous practice located in rural Minnesota, or upstate New York, or even next door in northern California. A practice is also a very personal business; it must be designed to accommodate the personal and professional needs and wishes of its owner. However, although practices may differ, their success is based on key features they have in common. This Guidebook will look at those key features and provide some pointers for planning your future.

Content

The Guidebook is divided into seven chapters that roughly follow a road from general information about the future of the mental health care delivery systems to highly specific suggestions for good business practices.

Changes in health care delivery have occurred at an alarming pace, and practitioners have had little time to carefully consider the direction of those changes and adapt to them. To set the stage for the business choices practitioners need to make, chapter 2, Environmental Assessment: A Look at the Health Care and Mental Health Care Marketplace, summarizes the much publicized problems in the U.S. health care sector, takes a quick look at some proposed changes, and examines the growth of managed care.

But long-range plans for mental health practices should not be made on the basis of today's environment alone. Chapter 3, Trends in Mental Health Care Delivery, identifies important changes affecting future practices of psychology.

In chapter 4, Models of Practice, the advantages and disadvantages of various forms of practice are explored. Many therapists who are practicing solo or in small groups are seeking ways to extend their capabilities by linking their services with complementary services of other providers, groups, or both. To assist the search for viable options, a variety of informal and formal organizations are examined in some detail.

No successful business—of any size—has become successful without good planning. Chapter 5, Developing Plans, leads the reader through a simple strategic planning process to the details of operational planning.

Chapter 6, Making Your Practice a Successful Business, lists the basic business systems that are needed to establish and operate a successful practice. Although it does not cover every contingency, standard policies and procedures are outlined. The chapter contains suggestions on improving business, administrative, communications, and other systems. Psychologists can choose those suggestions that fit their individual goals and objectives. Some useful forms, checklists, and guidelines are appended.

The Conclusion summarizes how the practice of psychology is being redefined and how psychologists can best cope with the changes created by that redefinition.

How to Use the Guidebook

The Guidebook is useful to practitioners in different ways depending on the maturity, size, and interests of the practices. It will introduce basic business concepts and help you ensure a professional, efficient practice. Chapters 2 and 3 establish a foundation for the practical suggestions that follow and should be of interest to all psychologists regardless of their form of practice. (The more practical chapters will appeal most to those who are relatively new to practice.) The planning chapter can serve as a refresher for those who are experienced in strategic planning or as a step-by-step process to be followed by others.

Chapters 2 and 3 provide the background for assessing opportunities and threats. Practitioners are recommended to read these chapters to get an overall view of the marketplace and the direction of future changes.

For those psychologists considering how to begin their practice or those considering changing their practice to meet marketplace demands, chapter 4 can help you decide about the most appropriate form to satisfy your personal and professional goals. Be sure to read this chapter before you contact an attorney to help you get started. By doing your homework, you will be better able to take advantage of his or her expertise. More experienced therapists should pay particular attention to the alliances that are described in this chapter.

Chapter 5 can be used as a practical guide for constructing a cost-effective business that provides high-quality services to your clients. For those practices that are operational, check your planning process and strategic plan against the one suggested here. Be sure to complete the appropriate forms in the Practice Analysis Tools in the Appendix so that you have the data needed to assess your strengths and weaknesses.

Chapter 6 has realistic, proven business techniques for many aspects of a professional practice. Although not all of the ideas will fit in every practice, the suggestions give you a foundation for choosing business practices and policies that will serve your practice now and in the future. Plan on returning to this chapter frequently in establishing your business procedures. Experienced practitioners should compare the business suggestions in this chapter with their current operations and adopt suggestions that will make their practice more efficient.

Although the Guidebook was not prepared as a business textbook, keep it handy on your reference shelf and refer to it when business questions arise in the operation of your practice. The book was designed to be leafed through again and again to find help for specific problems. Consequently, the Guidebook repeats itself regularly and duplicates related points or issues hoping to place the answer you seek where you can find it quickly.

You have already taken the first and most important step toward ensuring your practice's future success: You have recognized that you are not at the mercy of the forces that would discount your fees, limit the care you are allowed to give, and the living you are entitled to earn. Your practice is a business. And like any business, it must perform in order to compete in the marketplace. This manual will help you as you plan your strategies for future success.

2

Environmental Assessment

A Look at the Health Care and Mental Health Care Marketplace

The dramatic changes occurring in the delivery of health and mental health care services are forcing an examination of how practices are structured, how patients are referred, and how practitioners are reimbursed for their work. In the past, psychologists tended to be relatively independent—establishing solo practices, relying on former clients and colleagues for referrals of new patients, and receiving remuneration for services from third-party payers or directly from clients. The business aspects of providing services were simple; providers were free to concentrate on developing their professional skills.

The extraordinary rise of health care costs over the past two decades, which became an excessive burden on the purchasers of health care, has changed psychologists' sources of clients and income and is forcing a change in their primary mode of practice. These changes will continue to unfold. The forces of change discussed in this chapter include rising costs of health and mental health care, fragmentation of the system in which care is delivered, and questions about the quality of care. Reform of the health and mental health care system is also broadly discussed, with one particular attempted solution—managed care—viewed in some detail because of its widespread impact on the delivery of health care services.

Problems in Health and Mental Health Care

The problems associated with health and mental health care that have been discussed in most media sources have helped determine the outcome of national and state elections and have ultimately changed how Americans receive care. Each constituency, agency, consultant, or special interest group cites a different problem, including simple inflation, the cost of modern technology, unnecessary care, inefficient bureaucracies, risk-averse insurers, unscrupulous providers, fraud, and unwarranted malpractice claims. Although all of these contribute, three problems in particular—cost of care, access to care, and quality of care—are central to understanding the changes affecting the practice of psychology.

Cost of Care

The cost of health and mental health care is driving the call for reform. According to the federal government's Health Care Financing Administration (HCFA), na-

In $ Billions

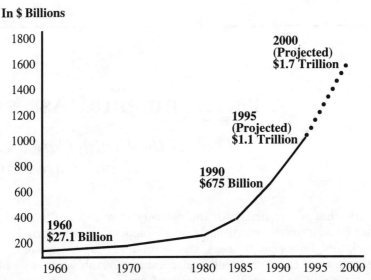

Figure 1. Health care spending projections. Health Care Financing Administration, 1993.

tional health care spending rose roughly 4,000% in the years spanning 1960 to 1990, when the nation spent $675 billion on health care. As can be seen in Figure 1, spending is projected to rise another 70% to $1.7 trillion by the year 2000.[1] Although recent cost data suggest that this trend is slowing, economists are uncertain whether it reflects a natural cost cycle, the effects of possible political reform, or the impact of managed care. Regardless, the cost of care is increasing faster than the general rate of inflation.

The dramatic cost increases of caring for an individual are borne by all sectors of the economy. For the federal government, total health care spending accounts for a huge portion of the overall federal budget—more than 17% in 1993. The impact on the economy is equally significant. As Figure 2 shows, approximately 12% of our gross national product (GNP) is spent on health care. This puts U.S. businesses at a significant disadvantage compared with their Western competitors, who typically have health expenditures of about 6% to 10% of GNP.[2]

These cost increases also have implications for the government's ability to fund major health and mental health care programs. Increasingly, health care programs are forced to compete with each other and with other federal program areas for scarce resources. Such programs include providing care to elderly and disabled individuals through Medicare, veterans and their dependents through veterans' benefits and the Civilian Health and Medical Plan of the Uniformed Services (CHAMPUS), and Native Americans through the Indian Health Service. In addition, the Medicaid program is charged with providing care to 28–30 million indigent Americans. This program, jointly funded by the federal and state governments, cost taxpayers $140 billion in 1993, representing a 100% increase over the last 4 years.[3]

[1]Sonnefeld, S., et al. (1993, Fall). Projections of health care spending through the year 2000. *Health Care Financing Review.*

[2]Sonnefeld, S., et al. (1993, Fall). Projections of health care spending through the year 2000. *Health Care Financing Review.*

[3]U.S. Department of Health and Human Services. (1992, December 31). *HHS Newsletter.*

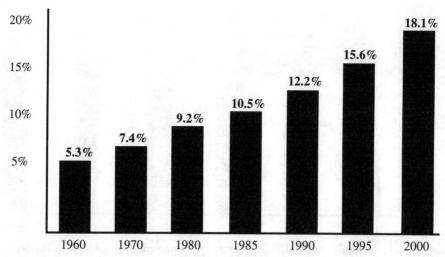

Figure 2. Health care spending (percentage of GNP). Health Care Financing Administration, 1993.

Each state also has the responsibility of funding public health programs, various categorical public health agencies, and providing health insurance to public employees and their dependents.

The private sector voluntarily assumes a major portion of the U.S. health care costs through provision of health insurance to employees and their dependents. Nearly 56% of the population has health care insurance through their employers. Business spent $205.4 billion on health services and supplies for their employees in 1992, or 28% of the total U.S. expenditure on health.[4] Because businesses ultimately bear much of the burden of paying for health care, any cost increase is of major concern to them. Between 1986 and 1993, the cost of employer-sponsored health insurance grew 3½ times faster than the overall rate of inflation and five times faster than wages for nonsupervisory workers.[5] As Figure 3 illustrates, the per employee costs for providing mental health care doubled between 1987 and 1992.

Many businesses have reacted to cost increases by passing them on to their employees. This strategy is known as "cost shifting." Through an increasing schedule of co-payments, deductibles, and other out-of-pocket expenses, consumers are paying for a greater portion of their health care services. Businesses today pay for approximately 69% of their workers' health care costs and workers pay the remaining 31%. By comparison, in 1970, businesses paid about 80% of the health care costs of their employees and dependents.[6]

---

[4]Health Care Financing Administration, Office of the Actuary. (1991). The report indicated that in 1991, $728.6 billion were spent on health services and supplies in the United States. Private business (public-sector employees were calculated separately) spent $205.4 billion on health services and supplies for employees. The cost included the employer's portion of insurance premiums, employer's portion of the Medicare tax, workers' compensation and temporary disability premiums, and industrial in-plant health services.

[5]KPMG Peat Marwick. (1993, November 30). Survey of 1003 firms. *Medical Benefits, 10*(22).

[6]Employee Benefits Research Institute. (1993, August). Survey reported in 1992. *The Health Care Consumer.*

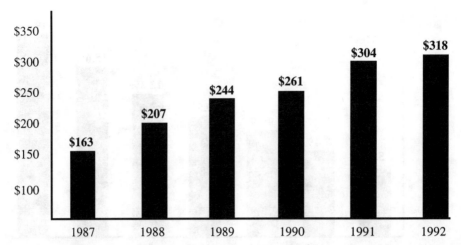

Figure 3.   Mental health costs (U.S. companies' average cost per employee). A. Foster Higgins, 1992.

When specifically considering behavioral disorders, treatment costs exceed $65 billion per year in the United States. The total impact of mental illness on the economy may exceed $270 billion when reduced productivity, mortality, and police and other law enforcement expenditures related to treatment of mental illness and substance abuse are added to the costs.[7] In recent years, expenses for substance abuse treatment and rehabilitation programs have increased exponentially, and the cost of mental health services for adolescents has risen rapidly. Many experts believe that a significant portion of this cost is due to inappropriate admissions to psychiatric inpatient facilities—the most expensive setting for treatment.[8] A number of studies have shown that as many as 75% of all patients admitted for substance abuse and 66% of all patients admitted as adolescents could be treated as effectively in outpatient settings.[9]

Access to Care

Cost is not the only pressing issue in today's health care environment. Many Americans do not have easy access to care. The U.S. health care system is based on health insurance as the primary method of payment, yet more than 37 million Americans do not have health insurance, which, in many cases, limits their ability and motivation to obtain care. Others lack access due to their remote locations. As a result, many Americans forego routine health care and ultimately seek treatment in more expensive settings such as hospital emergency rooms.

For mental health care, access to proper care is exacerbated by the reluctance

[7]Rice, D., et al. (1990). *The economic costs of alcohol and drug abuse and mental illness: 1985.* San Francisco: University of California, Institute for Health and Aging.

[8]Bacon, J. (1991). The challenges in mental health care benefits: Special report. What the experts advise. *Business & Health.*

[9]Strumwasser, I., et al. (1991, August). Appropriateness of psychiatric and substance abuse hospitalization. *Medical Care, 29*(8), AS77–AS90. Weithorn, L. A. (1988, February). Mental hospitalization of troubled youth. *Stanford Law Review, 40*(773), 773–838.

of many individuals to seek treatment and the inability of many in the medical profession to recognize the need for therapy and other health services. Access to continuing care is also seriously curtailed by the structure of mental health benefits offered by insurance companies. Insurance benefits for mental health services are significantly lower than those for physical health services, with limits on number of visits allowed and where treatment can be provided. Fully 94% of health benefits place some sort of arbitrary limit on outpatient mental health care.[10]

The decision to obtain health and mental health services is further aggravated by the choices and bureaucracy of care giving. Consumers often must determine for themselves where and how to seek services. Choices can be daunting: Services may be provided by public agencies such as the Departments of Public Health, Mental Health, Education, Justice, and Health and Welfare, or state and county mental health facilities, schools, or entitlement programs, and each may establish different criteria for obtaining services. Help may be provided by one's employer in the form of an employee assistance or health promotion program. Community activities sponsored by private, nonprofit mental health agencies or the support given by self-help groups add to a confusing collection of uncoordinated mental health services. It is not surprising that consumers may delay seeking treatment because of difficulty in selecting from among these options.

Quality of Care

Many purchasers of health and mental health care are concerned about the quality of care and question the efficacy of mental health treatment. Because purchasers generally do not understand the services being purchased, they tend to expect them to be comparable to medical and surgical services. That is, they expect to be able to devise the same sort of treatment guidelines and protocols and apply similar cost-control mechanisms for mental health problems as for physical health problems. Although the failure of these efforts is not surprising to mental health professionals, it confounds those without clinical experience. It contributes to the misperception that mental health care is less "scientific" than medical care.

Considering these factors as well as some negative portrayals of mental health care professionals in the media, it is not surprising that some observers have been led to question the quality and even the necessity of mental health care. As a result, in many states hospital licensure is now contingent on an institution's compliance with the standards set by the Joint Commission on Accreditation of Healthcare Organizations. And the National Committee for Quality Assurance's efforts to design a tool for evaluating health plan quality, the Health plan Employer Data Information Set (HEDIS) project, have kindled strong interest from businesses, the government, and consumers.

Efforts to Improve the Health Care System

There is no question that reform of the health care system is underway. The primary impetus for reform comes from those entities most feeling the pressure—federal

---

[10]*Business & Health.* (1993, September). Data watch: A sample of cost cutting strategies. 16–17.

and state governments, large and small businesses, and, to a lesser degree, consumers. This market-driven force for change takes a number of forms.

Government

Elections in 1992 at the federal and state levels helped to focus political attention on the problems in health and mental health care. The proposal offered by the Clinton Administration and the alternative plans promulgated by the Congress attempted to address the problems identified previously—containing the cost of care, improving access and coverage, and ensuring quality care—through a better integration of the delivery system. And although there are considerable differences among the bills about how these goals should be achieved, the overall goals are generally the same.

At least four major committees in the Senate and nine committees in the House will have jurisdiction over some part of health care reform legislation. And each committee will make changes in the legislation. It is virtually certain that the final House and Senate versions of the bills that emerge from the committees will be significantly different from each other. Reconciling the differences between the proposals will be the last major hurdle to health care reform and will, in all likelihood, redefine the structure of the American health care system. Changes resulting from national health care reform efforts will likely be phased in over several years.

As Figure 4 shows, state governments have also pursued reforms. Eleven states have passed major health care reform measures; nearly all are considering them.

Driven by the same concerns as the federal government, state initiatives take many forms:

■ Universal access: Although there are a number of strategies for providing universal access, the most common is through legislation that mandates employers, individuals, or both to purchase health insurance. Other strategies include expansion of the Medicaid program, managed competition, tax incentives, and

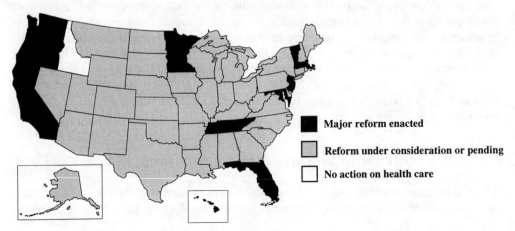

Figure 4.   State health care reform: 1993. APA Practice Directorate, 1994.

subsidies. New taxes may accompany universal access legislation to help cover the costs associated with providing care to more people.

- Employer mandates: Mandates generally require employers to offer and pay for a portion of their workers' health coverage. Hawaii and Washington currently have the only active employer mandates, and Massachusetts has passed a mandate that may go into effect in 1995.

- Single-payer and Multipayer systems: In a single-payer system, the government would collect premium dollars and administer benefits for covered residents. Insurance carriers would play a greatly diminished role. In a multipayer system, health care providers would be reimbursed according to guidelines established by a government agency. Vermont recently passed legislation designed to guarantee universal access via global budgeting, centralized planning, and insurance and malpractice reform. Montana and Colorado are also currently studying ways to adopt a single-payer or multipayer system.

- Managed competition: A number of states have enacted legislation on the basis of the principles of managed competition. Under this model, large health plans would compete with each other to deliver care to large groups of consumers. Minnesota, Florida, and Washington have all passed legislation intended to encourage managed competition arrangements.

- Health insurance industry reforms: Several states have taken steps to reform various facets of the health insurance industry. Legislation authorizing the creation of small group purchasing pools has been passed in a number of states (California, Texas, Minnesota, Vermont, Florida, New Jersey, Maryland, Connecticut, and Iowa). Because of their large size, purchasing pools are better able to acquire and negotiate fair prices for health insurance. Additionally, more than 40 states have adopted small employer or community rating laws designed to make insurance more affordable to small businesses.

Although hundreds of health-related bills were passed by state governments during the 1993 session, it is expected that even more bills will be enacted in 1994. Providers will need to be aware of the new state laws and their impact in order to survive as a business entity in the reformed system.

Corporate

Although federal and state governments have pursued legislative change, corporate America has demanded and pursued cost-control mechanisms. The private sector has been creative in developing alternative or innovative approaches to controlling the cost of health care benefits provided to their employees and dependents. Many have examined the delivery system for health and mental health care and elected to become more aggressive in changing their benefit design, contracting with managed care organizations (particularly those promising tight controls on spending), establishing their own provider networks by contracting directly with providers, and establishing employee assistance programs (EAPs) for administering mental health services.

Most employers attempt to direct their employees' consumption of health care services by carefully designing their health benefit programs. The use of incentives is one way to direct employees to services that the employer wants them to use. Another approach is attempting to select a network of efficient and cost-effective providers through a managed care organization (MCO) or through direct contracting and structuring the payment mechanism to reward employees for using those providers rather than out-of-network providers.

The concepts of managed care as a means of controlling cost have been widely accepted by businesses. Many firms insist on aggressive utilization review (UR) mechanisms, promote health maintenance organizations (HMOs) and preferred provider organizations (PPOs) to their employees, and design benefit packages that make consumers more knowledgeable about health care costs and more responsible for making appropriate choices about care.

Some employers have taken more control of their employees' benefits by contracting directly with a hospital or network of health care providers. Direct contracting has several advantages over traditional arrangements (e.g., an employer purchases health care through an insurance or managed care company). First, direct contracts do not involve an insurance "middleman," which lowers administrative costs. Direct contracts may also allow employers to take advantage of the value of specific services offered by a particular group or institution. And because federal law allows self-insured companies to design the benefits for their employees, direct contracting enables businesses to custom-make benefits. In many states, direct contracting relieves employers of the requirement to pay the per capita insurance tax required of standard insured benefit plans. As more sophisticated computer software makes it easier to manage and monitor direct contracting arrangements, this type of arrangement is expected to become more prevalent.

Some of the more successful measures emphasize prevention and early detection and treatment of disease. Wellness programs, EAPs, screening for disease and early prenatal care for employees or dependents help stem rising costs. EAPs also are typically able to act as a referral source for mental health services. Historically, the pathways for entering the mental health delivery system were referrals from physicians, clergy, teachers, or other professionals in the "caring" professions. Although EAPs were initially designed strictly to offer crisis intervention services, many have evolved into more full-service programs offering counseling and other forms of assistance to employees and their dependents who are experiencing stress, substance abuse, or emotional problems.

Another mechanism applied to mental health care has been the "carve-out," a behavioral health plan that is covered under a separate policy. Many of the mental health carve-outs include specialized inpatient and outpatient UR, a network of mental health and substance abuse counselors, case management, and claims paying and audit services that also credential providers. Typically, the entity that offers a mental health carve-out will have particular expertise in controlling costs in that area. In some cases, a managed care company is hired to administer the carve-out: select the panel of providers, conduct utilization review and other monitoring, and adjudicate claims.

Managed Care

One mechanism that promised greater control for purchasers was the replacement of traditional indemnity insurance plans with managed care. Managed care was

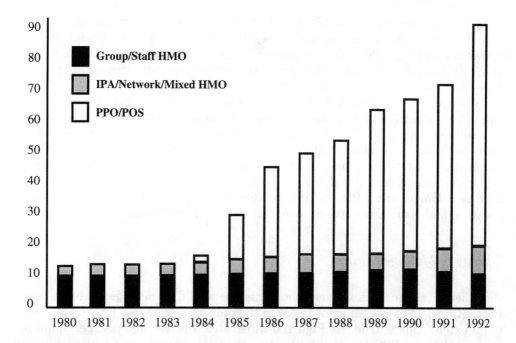

Figure 5. Managed care enrollment by type of plan: 1980–1992. GAO estimates based on data from Interstudy, KPMG Peat Marwick, and HIAA.

presented as the solution to the twin problems of lack of control over utilization and ever increasing costs.

It is important to understand what managed care is and what it is not. In this manual, an MCO is defined as an organization that provides a system of health care services to a predefined group of patients under a contract or on some basis different from traditional fee for service and manages the services provided to that group. The organization may include hospitals, physicians, therapists, laboratories, diagnostic centers, home care, and many other services.

In the classic example of an MCO, a panel of providers is selected that is willing to provide services for a predetermined, fixed price. Usually, services from these providers are fully reimbursable (up to the limits in the benefits plan) to either the patient or the service provider. When beneficiaries are permitted to choose a provider outside the panel, they usually are required to pay most, if not all, of the costs out of pocket. Thus, the health care purchaser—through the MCO's selection of providers—has considerable control over both cost and access.

Other forms of MCOs, such as PPOs, independent practice associations (IPAs) and point-of-service organizations (POSs) are growing in importance. Although some form of managed care has existed for several decades, little growth was evident until the 1970s. In 1980 only 9.7 million people were enrolled in HMOs; by July 1992 the number increased to 37.2 million (see Figure 5). The number of persons participating in managed care rises to 81.5 million when PPO participants are added.[11]

---

[11]Group Health Association of America. (1992, December 31). American Managed Care and Review Association. (1991, December 31).

Whatever their particular form, MCOs use a set of cost-control mechanisms, including UR, case management, the establishment of treatment guidelines, and outcome monitoring. Each of these mechanisms may take different forms depending on the MCO applying them. Their effectiveness consequently varies. Each is discussed in greater detail later in this manual.

Managed care is also changing as the health and mental health marketplace shifts. Pressures from their customers for greater cost containment and competition for enrollees among MCOs contribute to increasing numbers of mergers and acquisitions. One result of this activity is the formation of large, national networks of providers controlled by one organization and covering a significant number of lives. For example, traditional indemnity health insurers have purchased or formed their own HMOs and PPOs, which, in turn, have purchased hospitals, medical practices, and medical and psychiatric cost-management firms.

Efficacy of Managed Care

Many benefits managers in large companies believe that managed care has been and continues to be a significant factor in the reduction of overall health care costs. To an extent, this is true. As Figure 6 illustrates, the average cost per employee for an HMO or a PPO is significantly less than the average cost for enrolling an employee in a fee-for-service plan. Despite evidence that much of this difference in costs can be traced to other factors, the apparent difference in costs makes managed plans appealing to purchasers.

The achievements of the managed care industry need to be evaluated on a long-term basis and with some consideration for the effect on quality. Many long-term analyses show that managed care offers no real cost control and that much of the reported savings are the result of cost shifting and adverse selection. That is, younger, healthier people who generally have low medical costs choose managed care plans more frequently and thus account for lower utilization rates. The Government Accounting Office reported in October 1993 that "little empirical evidence exists on the cost savings of managed care. . . . Cost savings revealed in many studies may

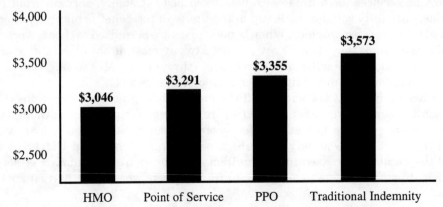

Figure 6. Average annual cost per employee by plan type. A. Foster Higgins, 1991.

be attributable to employee health status rather than to [actual] cost containment."[12]

An examination of the impact of managed care's methods for controlling costs on quality of care should give pause to those who embrace it as the solution to rising health care costs. Both the popular and medical literature are filled with reports of certain managed care entities improperly limiting patient access, causing treatment delays, censuring providers for giving quality care, and breaching patient confidentiality. Although it would be wrong to broadly condemn all managed care arrangements, it is clear that some managed care attempts to control costs have proved harmful to consumers. Moreover, cost savings continue to be elusive. Regardless, it is clear that some form of managed care is here to stay.

Summary

Responses to the problems in the health care delivery system, the influence of MCOs and their practices, and the increased interest of business in health matters have a direct impact on mental health practices. Clearly, the rise of managed care reduces the number of private-pay patients in the market and thus changes the market for mental health services. MCOs and employers are establishing regulations that providers must follow if they choose to treat the patients covered by these programs. In addition, the move toward organized networks of providers may make it more difficult to maintain a solo practice in the new marketplace.

External conditions—economic environment, health care reform by government and business, growth of managed care in response to the market, employer involvement, restrictions on benefits, and emphasis on outcomes—will have an impact on the long-range plans of providers of psychological services. The marketplace is reshaping mental health services. Buyers are seeking providers who understand business interests, operate like a business, and give an assurance of high-quality services at a competitive cost. Psychologists must consider how their practices will fare in the new environment. The remainder of this Guidebook offers the tools needed to take a proactive role in adapting your practice to the changes ahead.

---

[12]U.S. Government Accounting Office. (1993, October). *Report delivered to the House Ways and Means Committee* (Tech. Rep. No. GAO/HRD-94-3, B-254303).

3

Trends in Mental Health Care Delivery

The Corporatization of a Caring Profession

As major purchasers of health care in the United States, government and business are demanding greater control over health and mental health delivery systems. This fundamental reform, primarily based on the desire to control cost, shows no sign of slowing down. Some have called it the "industrialization" of health care; others have called it "corporatization" of health care—whatever the name, the result is the same. Providers of health and mental health care must be able to provide quality care, demonstrate the value of their services, and participate in an integrated, organized system.

The second chapter briefly discussed reasons for the shift in power from the caregiver to the purchaser. In this chapter, the implications of the shift—the "corporatization" of practice—are discussed by identifying trends in the mental health marketplace.

Trend 1: Mental health care is rapidly moving toward an organized, integrated system of care.

A vast array of programs, facilities, providers, and treatment options have left purchasers of behavioral health care services looking for ways to simplify decision making. In an effort to streamline their operations, they sought to contract with and fund a single system in which those in need of care can obtain necessary service. Such a system is "organized" because it integrates financing and delivery of care.

In this new system, psychologists will be selected on the basis of quality and cost management criteria. Ideally, the system uses continuous quality improvement processes and incentives to ensure that only appropriate and necessary care is given and is given at an appropriate intensity level (ambulatory, home care, hospitalization, etc.). The system is accountable to purchasers, patients, and others for cost, quality, and outcomes.

As streamlining intensifies, delivery systems will become horizontally and vertically integrated. The system will be vertically integrated when the services are organized and controlled by single organizations. For example, an MCO would own hospitals, clinics, and provider groups. On the other hand, if a particular health care system offers treatment in a range of settings by a range of providers, it is said to be horizontally integrated.

Trend 2: *To enhance leverage in obtaining contracts, practitioners are forming alliances and linkages with integrated systems.*

Becoming part of an organized system can be accomplished in many ways, including creating new entities, merging with existing practices, or developing linkages or alliances with other groups. A primary reason for any practice enhancement is to create a practice that is more attractive to purchasers; a single entity providing numerous services has a greater chance of obtaining a contract than do independent, unrelated practices. Such services would encompass full hospitalization, partial hospitalization, day treatment, and outpatient services.

Therefore, multidisciplinary groups and networks of practitioners are forming in order to increase their capacity for providing a full continuum of services cost effectively. For example, if some practices are composed entirely of clinical psychologists, they will position themselves with other practices that include social workers, psychiatrists, and physicians.

Geographically expanded practices are also being formed to serve buyers who are seeking comprehensive health services to cover consumers in many different locations. Established networks with practitioners in every region of the United States will be increasingly attractive to purchasers of care with interstate operations.

Trend 3: *Public- and private-sector systems are merging and moving toward a single system.*

Pooling public funds for health services with private-sector funds is expected to reduce the fragmentation of services and help control costs. Increasingly, public mental health agencies are contracting with private-sector groups to deliver necessary health care to the populations for which they are responsible. Consequently, they are downsizing their own staff. Proposed federal- and state-level reforms also provide opportunities for public and private health care services to be blended. At least 36 states are privatizing Medicaid or other health care programs for indigents in order to operate more efficiently and use public funds more responsibly.

In the future, psychologists will be reimbursed by different payers as needed (e.g., a health insurance carrier for one level of care and a public agency for another). To the patient and his or her family, the junctures between levels of care, the multiple service delivery sites, and funding sources will be nearly invisible because of the ease of moving from one setting or program to another.

Trend 4: *Corporate America's perception of psychologists has changed from providers of care to suppliers of a needed commodity.*

Until recently, mental health care represented a small portion of an employer's total health care costs. When utilization and cost rose dramatically, mental health benefits gained considerable attention from the business community. The cost of providing health care benefits has reached such proportions so as to be considered equivalent to any other costs of production. As a result, employers expect health care providers to conduct business in the same manner as other suppliers of goods and services. They want evidence of the quality of the product they are buying, competitive prices, and a long-term mutually beneficial relationship with the suppliers. They select mental health services on the basis of professional credentials, cost-effective practice methods, measurable positive outcomes, and business acumen. In short, business will demand better business from psychologists.

Trend 5: *Direct contracting between self-insured employers and mental health professionals is increasing.*

Buyers have learned that discounting the fees of providers, conducting utilization oversight, and collecting information on resource utilization can only go so far in reducing costs. To gain greater control over their benefits and cost, self-insured employers have begun contracting directly for health services with providers and facilities. This arrangement eliminates the insurance company middlemen, thus reducing administrative costs. Moreover, employers save money by self-insuring and may have direct control over the selection of practitioners.

Trend 6: *Purchasers and insurers are increasingly demanding financial risk-sharing with providers of mental health services.*

In the search for new cost-control mechanisms, health care purchasers are looking for new ways to regulate access and share financial risks. Increasingly, therapists are being asked to accept risk-sharing contracts. The primary risk-shifting mechanism is the provider payment system. In the past, the practice (or client) billed the insurer for covered services; the insurer assumed all financial risk. Insurers then began to contract for discounts on the providers' fees—shifting some risk to the provider. Fee-for-service arrangements nearly always include a discount, amount withheld for a risk-sharing pool, or both. A risk-sharing pool is a fund that accumulates the amounts withheld from a provider's fee according to a withholding arrangement. The pool is used to pay for any unexpected costs in the delivery of health care services. Discounted rates (or discounted fee schedules) are the least risky payment arrangement for the therapist because increases in the volume of service can compensate for lower rates. Often the amount of money in the withhold pool available for distribution is dependent on all practitioners operating in a cost-effective manner; thus, the purchaser's risk—and the risk of all members of the pool—is directly related to the selection of panel members.

Capitation, which is favored by some buyers, is the most risky payment arrangement for the practitioner. Under capitation, the therapist agrees to provide service to a defined population at an agreed-on price. Revenue to the provider is fixed by contract and not related to the number of individuals actually served in that population or the amount of care given to each individual.

Trend 7: *To achieve and sustain a competitive advantage, health providers are increasing their use of computer technology.*

Practitioners need ready access to information to meet the demands of the customers, measure effectiveness and efficiency, track contract arrangements and utilization, and stay current with research and practice. An information system powerful enough to fulfill these requirements must be computer based.

Traditional business applications are being adapted to suit practice needs. Electronic billing for services is growing rapidly; Medicare encourages computerized billing and most other insurers are building their capacity to use electronic billing. Legislation recently introduced by Missouri, Michigan, and other state legislatures supports a health care system electronic data interchange network that is designed to substantially reduce administrative costs.

Electronic record keeping has other major advantages, such as patient eligibility verification, treatment outcome analysis, and improved practice administration. In a fully integrated system of care, computers might be linked to provide patients' medical and social histories to psychologists (with appropriate controls for protecting the patient's right to privacy).

Effective management information systems store information about benefits, treatment, and outcomes that may be useful in advocating for changes in benefits. For practices involved in direct contracting or capitation, this information can be invaluable in negotiating new contracts.

Trend 8: *Practitioners are systematically measuring outcomes and building quality improvement systems.*

To control costs, large purchasers are attempting to select practitioners known to provide cost-effective care and who encourage the use of the most cost-effective treatment settings. Practitioners are recognizing the need to market directly to purchasers rather than only to the clients or consumers of their services.

Psychologists and physicians are developing standards of care and information systems to monitor adherence in order to market themselves as effective and quality health care providers. In the future, the standard for quality service will be defined by cost, utilization, prevention, and success as measured by practice guidelines and clinical protocols.

- Cost: In many cases, providers will be selected partly on the basis of cost profiles. Although the price charged for each service is relevant to this analysis, the systems will also evaluate the average cost per case of providers on the basis of data on the price and number of visits, length of treatment, and so forth.
- Utilization: Utilization of inpatient facilities and the prudent use of testing and evaluation procedures and other ancillary services will be another measure of quality. A practitioner will have his or her records compared with other providers to determine the average length of hospital stays for specific diagnoses, the degree to which each uses or does not use ancillary services, and whether colleagues or associate providers give service where appropriate.
- Prevention: Use of preventive measures and early interventions indicate qual-

ity health services. Preventing an illness or intervening in a stressful situation before it escalates is both less costly for the payer and less traumatic for the patient.

- Practice guidelines and clinical protocols: Practice guidelines and measurable clinical protocols that have been developed by mental health professionals, insurers, and patients will be used to assess the outcomes of treatment. Clinicians will be compared on their adherence to these guidelines and their percentage of successful clinical outcomes. This comparison will be used, in part, to determine which practitioners to include on provider panels. Mechanisms for evaluating individual or group performance with the objective of maintaining or improving the quality of care, often referred to as *peer review*, will become essential in mental health services delivery. The ability to demonstrate successful clinical outcomes on the basis of objective, professionally developed criteria will be a key factor in selecting service providers.

Trend 9: *To ensure a continuous flow of income, psychologists are diversifying their practices.*

Government reforms, corporate concerns over cost, the growth of managed care arrangements, reductions in benefits, and managed care mergers and acquisitions can radically reduce or even eliminate relied-on sources of revenue. If practice income is from one or a few sources, disruption may leave that practice without adequate sources of income. To sustain a financially viable practice, it will be necessary to have alternative sources of income. To diversify, practices may include a mix of income from the following:

- Teaching and research for businesses and universities
- Conducting behavioral assessments (for the school system, for clients of other therapists, for your own clients)
- Leading seminars for businesses, police departments, or other groups
- Participating in divorce mediation
- Giving expert witness testimony in child custody determination cases
- Concentrating on distinctive aspects of forensics
- Working with individuals who have medical conditions and their families (self-help groups of diabetics, candidates for surgical procedures, patients with terminal illnesses)
- Serving insurance and managed care companies as case managers, directors of quality improvement, and other managerial positions.

Summary

The corporatization of health and mental health care has a profound effect on the way psychological practices are organized. It is changing the way psychologists are viewed by purchasers of care, how care is delivered, and how practices are organized and operated. If psychological service organizations are to thrive in the projected health care environment, their practice and services will most likely be characterized in the following ways:

- Practitioners will be organized into horizontally and vertically integrated systems of care.
- Practices will include the full range of services or strong linkages to them and be able to refer clients to appropriate services; services will be integrated so that a clinical strategy for a patient can be carried out in a variety of settings as needed.
- Comprehensive services will be available even in remote geographical locations.
- Networks of providers will be multidisciplinary so that appropriate services can be provided through a single organization.
- Practice marketing plans will be designed for new audiences (large employers, MCOs, EAPs, etc.) as well as other therapists and former and current clients. Marketing tools will include data on outcomes and evidence of cost-effective practices.
- Practices will be business oriented using efficient, standardized procedures, accounting and other data processing systems, long-term strategic and operational planning, and productive marketing tools.
- Quality improvement and management systems will be used routinely. The monitoring systems that assess quality of care will include at least four factors: cost, utilization, prevention, and practice guidelines and clinical protocols.

Although these are significant changes, practitioners can adjust to the market conditions by becoming more business oriented without losing sight of their clinical and ethical mandates. The practice of the future must develop long-range business plans to ensure that it stays financially viable. Successful practitioners will see themselves not only as providers of care, but as proprietors of businesses in a competitive market.

4 _____

Models of Practice

Determining Which Type of Organization Is Best

With the changes in the health care arena and the rise of managed care, traditional models of psychological practice may no longer be advantageous in the marketplace. Much has been written about emerging or new models of practice—from groups without walls to multidisciplinary networks. However, determining which model of practice may be best is not a simple decision; many complicated and diverse factors contribute to that choice.

This chapter explores many of the factors that influence the choice of a practice model. A spectrum of models are identified, and their respective advantages and disadvantages are discussed; capitation arrangements are also briefly discussed. Furthermore, a chart that summarizes various legal organizations is included at the end of this section for your quick reference; however, it does not in any way constitute legal advice or direction. At the end of this chapter a supplement addresses the formation of a group practice.

One cautionary note: Not all models or combinations are explored. The specific needs of each marketplace vary greatly, and you should investigate the health care delivery environment in your area and be creative in choosing and developing the model of practice most appropriate for you.

Factors That Affect Choice

Choosing a form of practice is based on a number of factors: personal wishes that are often tied to a therapist's comfort with taking business risks and the degree to which autonomy and control is desired, consumer needs for "intimate" or "corporate" care, and market conditions, including the penetration of managed care into the marketplace. Also important are such considerations as legal structure and the needs of the purchaser of services.

Personal Preferences

Perhaps more than any other factor that may affect practice choice, your personal preferences are the most important. If your practice does not reflect what you wish to accomplish, you will not enjoy practicing psychology, and your practice will not be financially successful. In general, three sets of personal considerations are important when choosing a model of practice. You should examine the level of control available in that model (i.e., do you desire a great deal of autonomy over your practice and business?). Second, analyze your risk-taking capabilities (i.e., whether you need support from other professionals or desire a close, collegial relationship in your work and whether you are comfortable with taking business and financial risks). Finally, evaluate your desired level of income, including whether you need predictable income or whether you can tolerate swings in cash flow, whether you desire a great deal of leisure time, and whether the business plan you develop for your practice steers you toward one type of model. Conducting a thorough analysis of your personal preferences should be one of the first things you do when determining which model of practice is right for you.

Consumer Preferences

You will also need to gauge what consumer preferences are for the delivery of your services. In some communities, the solo practice is the most common model of practice, and patients are more likely to choose it for their care over other options. In other communities, purchasers may be directing their enrollees toward large, multidisciplinary groups. Before choosing a practice model, psychologists should inquire how other mental health professionals in the area have configured their practices and determine whether the market suggests that the current mode of practice should be continued. (For assistance in recording information from your analysis, see the Determination of Most Common Model of Practice worksheet at the end of this chapter.)

Market Preferences

Even though your preference may be to remain a solo practice, you may discover through a market analysis that a solo practice is not viable in your current locality.

You should examine the influence of managed care in your area. In some markets, a significant portion of mental health care is dictated by the purchaser of services—increasingly MCOs. Even if managed care is not presently a significant factor in the local market, you should investigate its rate of growth because it may rapidly become an influential force in the delivery of health services. There are several ways to conduct your review of managed care, but you may begin by reviewing the MCOs with whom you currently participate, speaking with your colleagues about the MCOs with whom they contract, and by calling the organizations directly to determine whether they operate or will be operating in your area. Moreover, it is likely that your state psychological association has relevant information on the influence of managed care in your area and any trends that may be unique to your state. (See Area Market Data worksheet at the end of this chapter.)

Legal Organization

Remaining in private practice will entail an examination of the legal issues that affect your selection of a model of practice. Most of the models of practice discussed in the previous section can be organized into any of the legal forms explored in this section. Four basic entities in which you may practice are presented: a sole proprietorship, a partnership, a professional corporation, or a limited liability company. These business organizations and their advantages and disadvantages are discussed; however, an attorney who is familiar with the relevant laws should be consulted before making any type of decision. You may also want to consult a financial or tax consultant to ensure that the form of practice you select meets your professional and personal financial goals.

Sole proprietorship. The least complex form of practice is a sole proprietorship, which is an unincorporated business owned and controlled by a single individual. In legal terms, there is no recognized entity separate from the proprietor. The therapist, as proprietor, owns all of the assets of the business and assumes all of its liabilities. In most states, all that is required to establish a sole proprietorship is for a psychologist to be licensed.

The advantages of a sole proprietorship are the simplicity of form and the business control afforded to you. A major disadvantage to a sole proprietorship is the risk of unlimited liability for all debts of the practice. Although most of the risk can be covered by insurance, creditors could seek liquidation of your personal assets to fulfill judgments against your business.

Partnership. A partnership is an association, governed by state law, of two or more therapists for the purpose of operating a psychological practice. The form is usually a general partnership, although some states may permit a limited partnership. In a general partnership, each of the partners is jointly and severally liable for almost all of the actions and debts of the partnership and the actions of all of the partners. That is, each of the partners is liable for the full amount of a judgment against a partnership; full satisfaction may be obtained from each partner or from a single partner. A limited partnership, however, reduces a partner's liability to the amount of the partner's investment, but it also restricts the involvement of a limited partner in the control and operation of the business.

In some states, partnerships can be formed on an informal basis; in other states, state law governs the formation, operation, and liabilities of a partnership. In either situation, it is recommended that an attorney prepare a formal partnership agreement in order to avoid future disputes. The agreement should cover all of the rights and responsibilities of the partners and delineate how the practice will be managed and operated. This document is designed as guidance for the partners in operating the business.

The major advantages of a partnership are the ease with which the entity can be formed and maintained, simplicity of operation, and that states typically require partnerships to file very little financial and other information with the state agency in charge of regulating partnerships. The principal disadvantage of the partnership model is the unlimited personal liability of each partner. In other words, you may lose personal assets such as a car or home when being held liable for partnership debts, even in circumstances in which you may have had no knowledge of your partners' actions. Liability for partnership acts could extend to malpractice claims, billing errors, and litigious conduct. Choose your partners carefully after a thorough discussion of professional and business issues and confirmation that you and your partners are compatible.

Professional corporation. A professional corporation or professional association is a legal entity separate from its practitioner-owners (shareholders). Although corporations are usually created by several individuals, a single practitioner can incorporate a practice. State laws strictly govern how professional corporations are formed and operated; although there are other types of corporations (commercial corporations, nonprofit corporations, etc.), all states require professionals who *deliver services through a corporate entity* to be organized as a professional corporation.

Professional corporations, similar to other types of corporations, must file articles of incorporation with the regulating agency of the state in which they operate. The articles of incorporation outline the purpose and ownership of the professional corporation, the shareholders, officers, directors, issues of stock, and so forth. Most states limit the shareholders and directors to a single profession, although some states permit psychologists and physicians to form professional corporations.

The corporation is governed by its articles of incorporation, bylaws, and shareholder agreements; these are legal documents that should be drafted by an attorney. After incorporation, a professional corporation must hold regular shareholder meetings, keep minutes, maintain corporate books, and generally follow the requirements of professional corporations in the state of incorporation.

The professional corporation is taxed as a separate entity. Retained earnings (profits) that are kept in the professional corporation at the end of the tax year are taxed at a corporate rate. Some professional corporations retain only minimal amounts at the close of the year and avoid double taxation by distributing earnings to shareholders (the distributions are dividends). Other professional corporations pay a salary to the officers of the professional corporation (the practitioner) and do not declare shareholder dividends.

One of the advantages of a professional corporation is the tax advantage it provides. A professional corporation, unlike a partnership or sole proprietorship, can typically deduct expenses relating to employee benefits. A professional corporation may also be able to deduct other expenses, and these should be thoroughly discussed with your attorney or tax consultant before forming a corporation.

Another main advantage of a professional corporation is the limited liability for shareholders and corporate officers. A shareholder or officer generally has no legal responsibility for satisfying the debts of the professional corporation, and a professional corporation structure usually protects your personal assets from the satisfaction of claims against the professional corporation. However, a professional corporation structure *does not* protect a practitioner from malpractice suits. A psychologist who is sued by the patient may be held liable for the full amount of the suit, and the psychologist's personal assets are not immune from judgment satisfaction.

The major disadvantages of a professional corporation are the more elaborate and somewhat costly formation and operation of the practice. There is also the possibility of being subject to both corporate and personal taxes.

Limited liability companies. A limited liability company is a new legal entity in which to form a business enterprise. Currently, 30 states have the limited liability company option available to entrepreneurs.[1] The limited liability company structure is a hybrid of a corporation and a partnership; thus, it has the advantages of both a corporate structure and a partnership structure.

The first advantage of a limited liability company is its limited liability for partners. Unlike a partnership, a partner in a limited liability company is liable only for the amount of the partner's investment in the limited liability company. That is, a general partner in a limited liability company does not have unlimited liability. The second advantage to a limited liability company is that all partners, in contrast to a limited partnership, may actively participate in management and operation activities. Consequently, a limited liability company is advantageous for heavily involved partners and "silent" partners.

However, there are disadvantages to a limited liability company. A limited liability company is taxed like a partnership; a partner pays taxes on his or her share of the limited liability company income regardless of whether the limited liability company declares dividends for shareholders. Furthermore, interests or shares in a limited liability company may not be freely transferred as in a partnership or a corporation. Rather, a partner in a limited liability company must fully withdraw from the enterprise and receive fair value for his or her interest. Consequently, a change in ownership in a limited liability company dissolves the existing enterprise and requires starting the formation process from the beginning.

Information on personal, consumer, and market preferences should be combined with the aforementioned discussion of legal organization possibilities and kept in mind as you explore possible models of practice.

Models of Practice

The models in which psychologists can practice range from the relatively simple solo practice structure to the highly complex networks of clinicians, groups, or both. In between these points lie a number of options for practitioners. In this section, the spectrum of options for psychological providers is explored by defining various models of practice, addressing how they are formed, and pointing out some of their advantages and disadvantages. The models presented in this section, however, are not exclusive and discrete; the various models may be combined and new ones created, or they may be diversified to fit your needs. The models in this section are simply a foundation from which to build the practice most suitable for your personal and professional goals.

Solo Practice

The solo practice is the least elaborate form of practice. Although it may have complicating nuances, a solo practice generally involves a psychologist practicing alone with additional staff as needed to handle administrative matters.

---

[1]States offering the option of forming limited liability companies are as follows: Alabama, Arizona, Arkansas, Colorado, Connecticut, Delaware, Florida, Georgia, Idaho, Illinois, Indiana, Kansas, Louisiana, Maryland, Michigan, Minnesota, Mississippi, Missouri, Montana, Nevada, New Mexico, North Dakota, Oklahoma, Rhode Island, South Dakota, Texas, Utah, Virginia, West Virginia, and Wyoming.

There are two major advantages to being a sole practitioner. A clinician in solo practice has a high degree of autonomy over the business (because there are no other clinicians involved in the decision-making process) and has fewer administrative burdens.

However, because of the complexities of the changing mental health care environment, it is becoming more difficult to operate a solo practice. Managed care companies that choose to do business with solo practitioners expect many of the same capabilities as they do from group practices. A partial list includes the following:

- Establishing a management information system
- Associating with other providers for peer support
- Instituting a sufficient call answering system
- Instituting quality assurance (QA) mechanisms and utilization review (UR) processes
- Conducting outcomes measurement studies
- Providing for inpatient care when necessary
- Undertaking risk-sharing mechanisms.

Solo practitioners are able to integrate all of these business systems into their practice, but they can be expensive and time consuming. Consequently, it is more difficult to conduct business with MCOs as a solo practice.

Other disadvantages to being a solo practitioner include unlimited personal liability, both legally and financially, greater financial restrictions, and greater limits on time and ability to manage both the practice of psychology and the business of psychology.

Informal Alliances

One way for solo practices to take advantage of the knowledge of others is to join or form an informal alliance. There are many ways to structure an informal alliance; it could be a group of providers who agree to meet once a week for peer supervision to discuss clinical issues, once a month to discuss business issues, or quarterly to discuss political issues affecting the practice of psychology. An informal alliance involves little, if any, financial commitment and little administrative commitment.

The advantages to an informal alliance are many. The main advantage is that an informal alliance allows practitioners to remain solo practitioners. Other advantages include an expanded referral base, at least minimal peer supervision, sharing office support, and a forum to vent your thoughts, suggestions, and frustrations.

The disadvantage to an informal alliance is that it is not a formal group practice. Legally, an informal alliance may not be perceived as a group or partnership. For example, if your informal alliance develops a logo for itself, you may give third parties the reasonable impression that your informal alliance is a group practice. Consequently, you may be held personally liable for your associates' behavior and debts of the informal alliance, without being able to take advantage of any protection you might receive from being a member of a formal group practice. Furthermore, you cannot market yourself as a group practice, and you cannot achieve economies of scale similar to a group practice. But, depending on your answers to the questions posed in this chapter, an informal alliance may be sufficient for your personal and professional goals. However, before undertaking any such endeavor, you should consult with an attorney who is familiar with these types of issues.

Formal Alliances: Groups and Networks

Certain conditions in your local market may demand a more formal organization of providers. If that is the case, then you should consider forming a group practice. A group practice consists of providers who have agreed to form a legal organization sharing facilities, records, and administrative staff and to practice together. A group practice involves investments of money and time into one legal entity and recognizing yourself as part of a group and the world recognizing your practice as one legal whole.

Furthermore, because of the changing health care delivery environment, group practices are more attractive to third-party payers. Mental health delivery systems are moving toward larger payers and networks. Because of the administrative ease of working with one group rather than several different practitioners, the economies of scale groups achieve, the ability to do "one-stop shopping," and a perception that groups are better at quality and utilization management, it is more efficient for these large payers and networks to contract with just one group of providers rather than several separate providers.

Group without walls. There are many types of group practices, and each type has its own costs and benefits. The first type of group is a group without walls (GWW). A GWW is a group practice, and a legal entity exists that recognizes it as such; however, the members of the group continue to work in their own offices. As a member of a group, you have access to more sophisticated office management services. As a group practice, a GWW has one body that makes management decisions, it may have a system to refer patients to the appropriate providers, its expenses are shared among the individual providers, and the entire group is responsible for any liabilities and debts.

One of the major advantages to a GWW is the ability to remain in an area where your practice is already established and avoid the costs of moving and leasing a new office. As a group, of course, a GWW can negotiate contracts with volume purchasers (MCOs, government agencies, etc.) that may greatly benefit each of the formerly individual practitioners. A GWW also expands your referral base because offices are more geographically dispersed (i.e., having 11 offices rather than just 3 offices increases the group's potential service area). A GWW can also be multispecialty, multidisciplinary, or both; you can be highly competitive if you are able to match your area of expertise with the market demands of the GWW area.

There are a number of drawbacks to GWWs. First, a GWW is a *group*, causing you to lose some of the autonomy you would otherwise have as a solo practitioner. In addition, forming a group requires reformulating your unique goals to the goals of a group. The goals you may have had as a solo practitioner will not necessarily be the same as the goals that a group will have. Because a GWW has many locations, it may also have hidden expenses from duplicated services or underutilized facilities.

Also, with a GWW there is a greater exposure to liability. In a traditional group practice, you may be responsible for the actions of your fellow associates, depending on the legal formation you choose. If you choose a legal entity such that you are liable for the actions of your associates, then it would be helpful to control those actions. That is much easier to do where you can see your associates on a daily basis and know what they are doing. It is more difficult when your associates are 50 miles away. Finally, a number of health care experts believe that the GWW mechanism has limited potential in a marketplace that is demanding more and more integration because the GWW is not integrated enough.

There are certain laws that prohibit referrals to certain health care providers: antikickback and antireferral laws. Thus, you must be especially careful when setting up a GWW's legal form and establishing its procedures. An attorney who is very familiar with antitrust and reimbursement laws should be consulted when forming a GWW.

Single-specialty group. Another option for practitioners who choose to be part of a group is a single-specialty group practice. This is a group practice composed of providers who practice the same type of psychology (e.g., industrial/organizational psychology, child psychology, or marriage therapy). Of all of the different types of groups, this is perhaps the least complex. A single-specialty group practice does not need to take into account factors other than the personalities of the various providers involved in the group practice.

Thus, one advantage of the single-specialty group practice is its simplicity. Furthermore, it may be easier to agree on clinical goals for the group if all of the group members have the same specialty. A third advantage to a single-specialty group is that it is legally easier to form a single-specialty group practice than to deal with the licensing laws of the various professions. However, a disadvantage to a single-specialty group practice is that it may become necessary to refer a patient to other practitioners or groups that have expanded capabilities. Depending on the marketplace, this may prove to be disadvantageous when contracting with MCOs, corporations, or EAPs. The single-specialty group practice may not have sufficient diversity to sustain itself in the evolving market.

Multispecialty group. A multispecialty group practice has as its members psychologists with different specialties. For example, a multispecialty group may include child psychologists, neuropsychologists, and substance abuse psychologists. This type of a group practice is slightly more complex due to the differences in specialties, but it holds many similarities to a single-specialty group.

The main advantage to a multispecialty group practice is the possibility of providing one-stop shopping for payers. A payor can contract with a multispecialty group practice and still receive the benefits of contracting with a wide range of practitioners. Furthermore, a multispecialty group practice offers stronger peer support, which is economically beneficial. A clinician in a multispecialty group practice can refer a patient to a different therapist in the same clinic; thus, not only is the patient benefited by receiving treatment from an experienced therapist, but the practitioner also receives the benefit of the patient seeing a therapist in the group and therefore augmenting group income.

The disadvantages of a group practice are amplified in a multispecialty group practice. Because of the different specialties, it may be more difficult to agree on clinical and professional goals. Furthermore, the different specialties also bring a broader mix of patients and administrative systems may need to be restructured in order to address this new dimension to client billing and record keeping.

Multidisciplinary group. The most complex model of group practice is the multispecialty, multidisciplinary group. In this model, psychologists with different specialties and different health professionals form a group practice. This type of group practice is the most attractive to payers because of the administrative conveniences of contracting with only one group and getting the full range of services. One-stop shopping for payers is the biggest advantage of the multidisciplinary group.

Furthermore, a multidisciplinary group requires less contracting with outsider providers. In states where psychologists do not have admitting privileges, this type of group often includes a psychiatrist, thus gaining access to inpatient facilities and reducing the potential for harmful and costly delays. Moreover, a multidisciplinary group including a psychiatrist also offers patients and payers prescription privileges that many psychologists do not have. And similar to a multispecialty group practice, referrals that are made to other therapists will most likely remain within the group, increasing both patient satisfaction and group income.

The major disadvantage to a multidisciplinary group practice is the level of complexity that this type of group entails. When there are many types of professionals in one group practice, billing and records must be integrated and centralized. Furthermore, the legal regulations affecting the formation of a multidisciplinary group may be more stringent, and, depending on the laws of your state, it may be impossible to form a multidisciplinary group practice without amendment to current laws governing the incorporation of professionals. You should consult with an attorney experienced in health care organizations when deciding whether to form a multidisciplinary group practice.

In addition to the group practice, there are other formal alliances in which providers may build their practices. These alliances are called "networks," and they include management services organizations (MSOs), provider–hospital organizations (PHOs), PPOs, IPAs, or HMOs. There are advantages to either joining a network or to forming a network, but state and federal regulation may make forming a network expensive and difficult.

Management services organization. An MSO is an entity that is usually jointly owned by several practitioners created for the sole purpose of providing management services to each of the participating practices. The MSO is a legal entity separate from the individual practices. As such, it can have assets and liabilities and can represent its members in the marketplace in limited circumstances. The MSO conducts the administrative and management functions that are desired by the therapists who participate. Therapists pay a fee to the MSO for services that might include billing services, insurance claims processing, and collections. The principals do not become employees of the MSO, and income is not co-mingled. The participants determine the scope of services provided by the MSO and establish its management procedures.

MSOs and their participants must be aware of antitrust regulations that prohibit them from jointly establishing prices or from refusing as a group to deal with payers.

Provider–hospital organization. A PHO is a "merger" of providers and hospitals, with the final entity being jointly owned by the providers and the hospitals. As with a multidisciplinary group practice, a PHO allows providers and hospitals to operate as a single organization that provides a wide range of health care services, thus being more attractive to payers.

Two key issues involving PHOs are financial. The hospital will have access to more capital, but providers are also expected to contribute to financing the venture. Furthermore, how revenue will be allocated is important. The PHO is likely to engage in capitation arrangements and then either pay providers on a fee-for-service basis or capitation basis as well. Because PHOs are new entities, it is particularly important for you to consult an attorney when considering the PHO structure.

The advantages to a PHO include the ability to provide an integrated system of services and increased bargaining power with respect to payers. However, some MCOs prefer to contract with providers independently, and a PHO structure may actually deter some MCOs from contracting with you. Furthermore, PHOs may lead to tension between the provider and the hospital over control of the delivery of services and to conflicts with professional goals. Yet, PHOs are considered by many to be the state of the art in integrated delivery systems.

Preferred provider organization. A PPO is an organization formed, usually by large health care and insurance companies, to provide a package of mental health services to purchasers. The buyers of the PPO arrangements give their employees and enrollees incentives to use the PPO providers rather than non-PPO providers who might charge a higher fee.

Typically, PPOs serve as "go-betweens." They determine what benefits and incentives purchasers believe will encourage their members to use PPO providers. The PPO then contracts with therapists to join the PPO and provide those benefits. Each therapist who joins a PPO signs an agreement to provide services at the lowered rate, and, in many cases, the PPO provider agrees to abide by other rules regarding UR procedures or balance billing to patients.

In joining a PPO, providers usually agree to discount their fees in exchange for an increased volume of referrals. Other advantages to joining a PPO include increased peer support, an entity that can serve as the representative for your services, and practitioners can maintain their solo or group practice status while participating in a PPO.

Joining a PPO has some disadvantages. First, a PPO does not guarantee increased future referrals. Thus, a provider may discount his or her fees and not have sufficient patients to offset that discount. Second, a PPO is an MCO that may be primarily concerned with cost containment. Consequently, a PPO may entail UR, case management, confidentiality problems, and numerous other difficulties.

Although it is possible to start a PPO, forming one is a major enterprise in many states because there may be laws controlling the formation and operation of PPOs. In states that regulate PPOs, requirements often include offering both medical and mental health benefits, contracting with a large variety of providers, and developing comprehensive enrollee information materials. These types of specifications for PPOs often render forming a PPO unrealistic for many practitioners. However, if forming a PPO is the appropriate option for meeting your professional and personal goals, you should first consult with a health care attorney who is familiar with the managed care and insurance laws in your state and with state health care reform as well.

Health maintenance organizations. HMOs are managed care entities that combine the insurance of health care services with the delivery of those services. Because HMOs act as insurers, it is highly improbable that most practitioners have the financial resources to build an HMO. However, either as a solo or group practice, it is quite feasible for you to join an HMO as a network provider.

The advantages of joining HMOs are that some HMOs employ their providers, giving a practitioner financial security and increased referrals. Because HMO enrollees may see only HMO providers in order to receive coverage for services, the practitioner is almost guaranteed an increased number of patients.

However, HMOs also contract with providers to deliver services on a discounted basis. Discounts that are negotiated with providers are sometimes so low that many providers drop out of the panel. Furthermore, the financial incentives offered to providers can encourage and often lead to underutilization of services.

Independent practice association. The fastest growing type of HMO is the IPA-model HMO. In an IPA, independent practitioners form a new entity in order to contract with volume buyers. Typically, an IPA is paid a capitated rate by an HMO for the services that are offered by the IPA; the IPA, in turn, contracts with providers who are usually reimbursed on a discounted fee-for-service basis or a capitated rate basis. If the clinicians are reimbursed on a fee-for-service basis, then a specified amount is usually withheld in a risk pool. If the cost of services is less than anticipated, then the money in the risk pool is distributed to providers. If the cost of services is more than anticipated, the risk pool is used to cover those extra expenses and the providers forfeit that amount. Because an IPA involves capitated fee arrangements, forming this type of an organization is usually undertaken by practitioners with business experience and large amounts of capital. For solo practitioners and small group practices, joining an already established IPA as a network provider may be a much more feasible option.

An increased number of managed care companies are seeking to share the risk of delivery of services with providers. The most common way to do this is through a capitated fee structure, but providers are reluctant to accept risk. An IPA allows practitioners to accept risk such that they are able to reap large gains but are protected against large losses. Furthermore, an IPA also allows practitioners to retain their solo or group practice status while being a member of an IPA; many practitioners continue to see non-IPA patients while seeing IPA patients. However, IPAs may be subject to state laws similar to HMO laws. You should contact an attorney in your state before forming an IPA.

Furthermore, there may be an incentive to underutilize services because providers may be responsible for unanticipated costs in providing services. An IPA can be structured so as not to encourage providers to place financial considerations ahead of clinical considerations.

Capitation

Many of the models of practice discussed thus far are well positioned to pursue "capitated" reimbursement arrangements with large purchasers of mental health services. In recent years, many private and public purchasers of health services have embraced capitated health systems as a means of better controlling health costs. This approach is rapidly increasing in popularity, but such agreements need to be carefully crafted. The actuarial counsel of an experienced risk adjustor who is familiar with local utilization patterns is recommended if not essential.

Broadly speaking, capitation is a payment agreement for a package of health services on a prepaid basis per enrollee without regard to the actual frequency, extent or kinds of services provided. The amount of a capitated arrangement is calculated on the basis of the expected utilization of services for the covered population. The essence of capitation—and the reason for its attractiveness—is the transfer of significant financial risk from the purchaser of services to the deliverer of services.

Capitated arrangements may be either "community rated," where the payment for each member of the group is presumed to be the same, or they may be calculated on an "adjusted" (also called "experience-rated") basis, in which members of a group are rated differently to take into account various demographic factors or other predictors of service utilization (e.g., employment setting, disability status, local economy, institutional status, etc.). These demographic and other factors are extremely significant in determining the utilization of mental health services.

In pursuing a capitated agreement for the provision of mental health services, the following elements should be given serious consideration:

- To develop cost estimates that are as reliable as possible, significant historical databases are needed to establish expected utilization patterns. These estimates must, however, be adjusted according to local conditions, specific covered populations, any nonstandard utilization patterns, or other relevant factors.
- Large numbers of capitated individuals are necessary in order to achieve an adequate spreading of risk. If sufficient volume cannot be realized, other reimbursement approaches (e.g., per-case rates) should be pursued.
- Mental health providers should be able to significantly control referrals to inpatient facilities and to other types of health care providers. If inappropriate referrals cannot be controlled, capitated arrangements are far less likely to be successful. Teamwork and an integrated delivery system are essential components of a capitation contract, as are establishing parameters for dealing with difficult cases. It is important that provider and payer share the same treatment philosophy.
- The scope of services must be rigorously defined.

- Actuarially sound risk adjustments specific to the relevant local area (or areas) must be developed, incorporating demographic differences, health status, occupation, industry, and so forth.
- Providers should always be shielded against unexpectedly high utilization rates. This can be accomplished through the use of individual stop-loss agreements or reverting to a fee for service arrangement for excess utilization from certain patients.
- Any financial incentives should be designed to reward both efficiency and quality. Performance requirements should be understandable, measurable, and equitable for the providers. Performance requirements must also take into account the severity of illness of the treated patient population. Performance appraisals should be used constructively, rather than punitively, in order to help improve provider effectiveness.
- Administrative and management information systems are needed for utilization reporting, accounting, referral tracking, UR, and billing.

Although there is no standard formula for calculating the estimated costs for providing inpatient and outpatient services to a given population, the following example may be used as a framework for estimating costs. It is important to remember this is only an example. The utilization and cost figures which are presented in this example **should not be used for calculating a capitated arrangement in your location**. Utilization patterns, treatment approaches, and costs will vary considerably from contract to contract and practice to practice. This model identifies only the basic information you must examine in order to pursue a capitated arrangement; other significant factors that may affect costs (medical management, crisis services, etc.) are not accounted for. This model is based on a contract for 100,000 covered lives.

Example

I. Outpatient Utilization

3% per 1,000 lives	3,000 patients
Averge # of visits	9 visits
Average cost per visit[a]	$76
Outpatient provider cost	$2,052,000

II. Inpatient Utilization

23 days per 1,000 lives	2,300 days
Average length of stay	11 days
# MD visits	1,840
Total cost of MD visits	$174,800
PhD testing of 65% of admits	approx 250 patients
Average cost of testing	$400
Total testing costs	$100,000
Total MD and PhD costs for inpatient delivered care	$274,800

III. Overhead costs[b]

	Monthly costs
Total supplies, rent, etc.	$48,000
Total Overhead per year	$580,000

IV. Total Cost for Arrangement

(Inpatient Cost + Outpatient Cost + Overhead)/Number of lives covered by contract/12 months = Capitation cost per life per month

($274,800 + $2,052,000 + $580,000)/100,000/12 = $2.42 per person per month

---

[a]The average cost per visit may be calculated by determining the cost for each type of provider (PhD, MD, MSW), multiplied by the average number of visits (by provider), multiplied by the expected number of patients seen by each provider type. Add these three totals and divide by the total number of expected outpatient visits.

[b]More is said about figuring out overhead costs in chapter 6, Business Strategies. Example is based on the assumption that overhead will amount to roughly 25% of the cost of services provided.

Of course, a suitable profit margin is always factored in as well. This is not reflected in the example above. It is important to remember that additional information such as locality, patient population, education, age, treatment approach, and the use of different professionals will all significantly affect the overall cost of providing services.

Markets for Your Services

Once you have chosen the model of practice, you should also examine the various markets for your services.

Local Employers

Self-insured employers often select their own panel of therapists with whom to work. Contractual arrangements may be made directly with the employer or a company-sponsored EAP. Employers who carry mental health care insurance for their employees may recommend you to the carrier or the MCO that is handling their benefits.

Employers may be willing to subcontract for some or all of their outpatient mental health services. How much you can undertake will depend on the size of your group and the depth of its experience. For mature, experienced organizations that are capable of risk sharing, you may elect to carve-out both the inpatient and outpatient mental health benefits on a capitated basis. Be sure that someone experienced in negotiating risk-sharing contracts assists you with these arrangements. For new groups, you may decide to work through an informal collaboration; for example, you may consider working directly with the EAP or human resources staff to obtain referrals.

More and more employers and psychologists are choosing to work directly with each other in order to overcome the deficiencies of managed care. This arrangement eliminates the middleperson, thus reducing administrative costs and giving the employer more control over the delivery of benefits.

Managed Care Organizations

HMOs, PPOs, and other MCOs maintain panels of providers with a depth of expertise and a broad range of skills. Practitioners may find that these purchasers are seeking additional panel members with your skills. This may be a particularly attractive option if you or your group has an expertise in a specific area of practice.

You can petition to become a member of an MCO panel. Before approaching an MCO, you should conduct some research on the organization. Determine what types of providers it is seeking, in which location it does not have many psychologists, and its treatment philosophies. You should also contact your state psychological association because it may have gathered data on various MCOs. Once you have investigated the MCOs that are most appropriate for you, you should prepare the following documents to accompany your letter of petition:

- Your credentials (curriculum vitae)
- Practice data (e.g., types of cases you handle, the average number of visits per type of case, average length of inpatient treatment, cost per case, etc.)
- A statement about your mental health treatment philosophy
- A description of your initial patient evaluation process
- The results of patient satisfaction surveys or other measurable outcome data
- References from other professionals in your referral network.

The Practice Record and Staff and Services portions of the Practice Analysis Tools (PATs) in the Appendix can be used to organize your letter of petition. A letter of petition that incorporates a reasoned analysis of many of these items will be particularly useful in approaching MCOs that have otherwise closed their provider panels or are reducing the number of providers with whom they contract. In the event that you are turned down, do not be afraid to be persistent. Securing a spot on an MCO panel may be a matter of continuing negotiation and demonstrating the ability to successfully "sell" the MCO on your services.

Some MCOs enter into employment relationships with their providers. Although employment is usually with a staff-model HMO, other MCOs may offer full- or part-time employment. For individuals who prefer regular hours, stable income, and few management and business responsibilities, this could be an attractive arrangement.

Employee Assistance Programs

EAPs were originally created by employers to deal with employees' substance abuse problems, but they have expanded to cover a wide range of health services. Internal EAPs are directed and managed by company staff with additional therapists as contract employees. External EAPs contract with individuals, groups, social service agencies, and others to provide resources. External EAPs often serve the employees of several employers in the community. Usually, an on-site EAP staff member determines where employees or their family members will be referred. In addition to providing direct services to clients referred by EAPs, psychologists may consult on the development of the company's mental health policies, health promotion and disease prevention activities, and strategies for stress reduction activities.

Primary Care Physicians

Primary care physicians (PCPs) have become more prominent in the health care scene of the 1990s than at any other time in recent memory. MCOs place great responsibility on PCPs to provide the bulk of medical care to their enrollees and to determine if and when referrals to specialists are appropriate. These physicians are in a position to refer patients to psychologists for a variety of preventive care and therapy.

According to a report in the *Journal of the American Medical Association*, PCPs have difficulty diagnosing mental disorders in patients who have them.[2] This is not surprising because PCPs are not specially trained to recognize and diagnose mental illness. But consequently, many patients do not receive the mental health care they need. Working collaboratively with PCPs in your area would provide them with valuable assistance in recognizing mental illnesses and provide you or your group with new sources of referrals.

Summary

The models for mental health delivery are many and varied, yet none will meet all of the requirements of every practitioner. Choosing the best model is difficult, but the choice is not irrevocable. As market conditions change, practices mature, and alliances shift, the model chosen can be reconsidered and a new choice made. What is important to remember is that you are in control of this choice, and the information presented in this chapter will aid you in making that choice.

---

[2]Wells, K. B., et al. (1989). Detection of depressive disorder for patients receiving prepaid or fee-for-service care. *Journal of the American Medical Association, 262,* 3298–3302.

Chapter 4
Supplementary
Materials

Forms of Legal Entities in Practice

	Organization	Legal Structure	Termination	Advantages	Disadvantages
Sole Proprietorship	Owned by one practitioner	No grant or charter from the state required	Upon death of proprietor	Minimal cost and ease of formation Sole management responsibility Simplicity of operation Flexibility Minimal reporting requirements	Sole management responsibility Unavailability of many employee benefits Unlimited personal liability for debts and actions of the business and its employees
Partnership	Owned and managed by two or more persons	Partnership agreement Other requirements as specified by state law	Dissolution upon death, withdrawal, bankruptcy, or insanity of any of the partners	Minimal cost and ease of formation Centralized or shared management Simplicity of operation	Centralized or shared management Unlimited personal liability for debts and actions of partnership Unable to deduct costs of many benefits Possible unlimited personal liability for misconduct of partners and staff

Professional Corporation	Considered by law to be a separate legal entity One or more psychologists may be a professional corporation	Professional corporations must comply with all requirements set out by state law. Unless otherwise specified by state law, all members of the professional corporation must practice the same profession	The bylaws of the professional corporation should specify circumstances for liquidation and have provisions for the buyout of a shareholder	Limited personal liability for debts of corporation Can deduct cost of benefits Centralized or shared management Free transferability of ownership by stock distribution Estate planning and insurance planning opportunities	More costly formation May have centralized or shared management More formalities of compliance Double taxation on corporate and shareholder income Remain personally liable for professional judgments against oneself and, in some states, against other shareholders
Limited Liability Company (LLC)	May be formed by two or more persons	Hybrid between corporation and partnership. Separate state laws govern the formation of LLCs	Partner may buy out of LLC or as specified by state law	Limited personal liability for partners All partners may participate in the operation of the business, regardless of their investment	Interests in LLC may not be freely transferred to other persons Not available in all states

Note. This chart does not in any way constitute legal advice or direction.

Determination of Most Common Model of Practice

The purpose of this worksheet is to capture some information that will help you decide if there is one form of practice that occurs more often in the local community. To gather that information, try some of these methods.

- Call the psychological association (local or state) to ask for information about the forms of practice of their members.

  _____

  _____

  _____

- Skim the telephone Yellow Pages. Make a rough count of those listings that appear to represent solo practitioners and those that are groups or clinics.

  _____

  _____

  _____

- Call five or six of your colleagues (or randomly select some psychologists listed in the telephone directory) and ask their perception of the most common form of practice.

  _____

  _____

  _____

- Call the psychologists' referral services listed in the Yellow Pages and discuss with them the primary form of practice represented by their service. Ask the same question of staff at local psychiatric hospitals.

  _____

  _____

  _____

- Call the MCOs in the community (ask for a case manager) and determine their view of the local market.

  _____

  _____

  _____

Although these techniques rely on personal opinions and other "soft" data, the findings are still valuable to you in making your decision about a form of practice. If all of the therapists in your community are practicing solo or in very small groups and you are interested in forming a large multispecialty practice, you will know that you may have some selling to do to get others interested in your plan. However, if you also want to open a solo practice, you will know that model is acceptable and known in the area.

How to Form a Group

The formation of a group—no matter how informal—takes time, effort, and money and the decision to begin one should not be taken lightly. The steps below are easy to list but much more difficult to execute. There is no template that you can follow to assure success. The successful formation of a group requires commitment from its leaders, who will need to take the following steps.

- Develop a statement of purpose. State clearly why this group should be formed. This statement of purpose will be used frequently to orient and recruit potential group members.
- Decide what services and activities will be performed by the group. Be specific about the types of health services that will be included, how the group will market its products, and for whom it will provide services. Early in the formation, the group must face the credentials of membership, how cost and quality will be measured, and whether therapists who do not measure up to the standards set by the group will be dropped.
- Prepare a business plan. After identifying the business operations that will be included in the group, list the resources that will be needed. Include human resources as well as physical assets. An important part of the business plan is the market assessment and projections of the portion of the market this group can capture—and when. Put together a budget that includes the cost of start-up, initial operating expenses, and the estimates of ongoing revenue and operating expenses.
- Decide who will be the owners of the group. The group has many options, and each has implications for growth and for its finances. For example, the founders can be the sole owners and other therapists can be added as employees. This model requires significant investment from the founders or perhaps slow growth due to lack of capital. If each therapist who joins the group becomes a part owner, the group can require that each contribute some capital. Be sure to check with your attorney or other advisor to be sure that there are no legal requirements to be considered.

Assuming that these first steps have been performed to the satisfaction of the group leaders, the next steps involve legal and regulatory issues. Obtain experts—both legal and management consultants if necessary—who have had experience in the formation of groups similar to the one that you are planning. (See the section on choosing and using consultants, which appears at the end of chapter 6.)

- Determine the legal structure of the group. Review the antitrust implications in the group before you decide on the size of the group and the price determination process.
- Establish the ongoing governance structure. Although the leaders during the formation may be good choices for the initial governance, the group needs to define the governing board's composition, the limits of authority for managers and board members, and decide on voting rights and bylaws.
- After the governance structure has been resolved, the group may need to check

on regulatory issues that apply to the structure and governance of the group. For example, in some states the formation of a PPO or IPA would require compliance with insurance regulations.

■ As with any organization, the creation of a group requires the preparation of several documents that establish the existence of the group and the legal relationships with its members. After your attorney has drafted all of the documents, the psychologists should review the documents and be assured that they represent the intentions of the owners and members of the group.

5

Developing Plans

Assessing Your Situation and Taking Action

When you completed your professional training, you probably felt well prepared to provide caring, patient-oriented therapy, were comfortable with your competency level, and looked forward to meeting the demands of working with clients. You may have been imbued with the idealism that is often part of the atmosphere in academic centers.

However, then you faced the realism of operating a business. Nothing in your professional training had prepared you for selecting accounting systems, contracting with service organizations, or dealing with the myriad problems of setting up a new enterprise or deciding which practice held the best business opportunity as well as the best professional opportunity for you. Or you may have been disinterested in being an entrepreneur and wished that you could order a ready-made practice so that you need not be bothered with business concerns.

The most effective way to overcome the discrepancy between what you were educated to do and the business operations that you must do in order to use your education is to develop a business plan. When the steps of putting together the business side of your practice are defined, you may be surprised at how much you know about running a business. This chapter covers the business planning that is inevitable regardless of what form of practice you choose.

Unfortunately, there are no blueprints that you can use to develop a business as personal as the practice of psychology. You can look at someone else's practice model to gain ideas, but you would be foolish to implement another's plan. Take the time to systematically design your own professional life. The first move should be to review all of the opportunities available to you. Whether you are just beginning or are already in practice, take a look at the old and new options.

Assessment

To prepare for examining some opportunities, you need to conduct two analyses: internal and external. The Practice Analysis Tools (PATs) that appear in the Appendix offer an excellent way of capturing all of the information that you need for these analyses. Not all of the questions can be answered by facts. Some of them address your personal feelings and professional goals.

Practice Analysis

- From the PATs in the Appendix, complete the Practice Record, a description of your practice, and a Fact Sheet pertaining to your credentials and services. Later, you should request fact sheets from all of the therapists in your practice for a better view of the expertise of the entire practice.
- Think about your personal preferences for your practice—the internal part of the assessment. Do you prefer to have control over your hours of work and your personal time? Are you interested in other aspects of your profession such as teaching or research that create conflicts with seeing patients? How invested are you in building a career?

  Do you want to limit your practice to certain types of cases or diagnoses? Would you prefer to carry a smaller case load (and have a lower income) in exchange for being able to choose your clients? Do you want to pursue excellence in a particular, but narrow, aspect of mental health treatment?

  To what extent do you want to become personally involved in business management? How strong is your interest in retaining control of your practice? Are you interested in learning more about computers, accounting, and health insurance? Would you like to help form a group or alliance of other therapists?
- Complete the Referral Data Form, Patient–Payer Profile, and Business Management sections of the PATs. If you do not have access to the information, guess at the answers. You will want to verify your guesses before you make concrete plans, but impressions are enough for now.
- Looking at your patients, referral base, and financial status, how viable is your practice? Can you continue in your present mode of operation for the foreseeable future? Do you have enough patients to withstand changes in insurance coverage that might force your sources to refer elsewhere? Are your sources of patients diversified?

  Are your overhead costs reasonable? Are you performing many nontherapy tasks yourself? Do you get a reasonable collection ratio (85% or higher of what you bill)? Are you interested in a stable income? Do you want to plan for a high-volume, high-income practice?

Environmental Analysis

- If you have not already done so, complete the Area Market Data form mentioned in chapter 4 and located in the PATs for a look at the business and health care environment.

  What percentage of the market in your community is committed to managed care? How does your managed care patient load compare with the market? For example, if the local market share for managed care is 28%, is your income from MCOs less or more than 28% of total income?

  Are EAPs and private employers contracting with individual therapists for the care of their enrollees or employees? Are there too few, too many, or just the right number of practitioners in your area? Are there shortages in a particular specialty?

In addition to the data that you have collected about your practice and recorded on the PAT forms, you may want to discuss some of these questions with your accountant or other business advisors. If you meet regularly with other therapists to discuss business matters, the external assessment questions might be raised at those meetings so that you could have the benefit of their analysis.

Interpretation

As you well know from your clinical training, the assessment just completed is not very meaningful until the data are interpreted. Look for clues that provide direction. For example,

- Do you see a strong entrepreneurial bent to your responses? Interest in the business aspects of practice might lead you to consider solo practice or a group in which you could assume a management role.
- Are your responses skewed toward building social and collegial relationships through practice activities? Do you favor a varied practice treating many different types of cases? If yes, a multispecialty group or employment in an agency with many services might be the most appropriate.
- Does your analysis of the community show that managed care is greater than 40% of the market? Are there numerous large employers in the area? If so, you might consider the protection from capricious market swings that a group practice affords. Or you could pursue the formation of a PPO or IPA to gain market leverage.
- Does the snapshot of the environment reflect a traditional community in which most of the common forms of practice exist? Are the traditional forms of insurance equally represented in the patient population? If so, solo practice, small groups, or informal alliances might be the most appropriate practices to seek.

Practice Options

The purpose of any assessment and interpretation of data is to determine whether changes need to be made. These changes might be based on personal, professional, or financial needs. The assessment that you just completed should point to one of the following options.

- After assessing your current practice or your newly acquired education as a therapist, personal preferences, and the local market conditions, you may decide to establish or remain in a solo or small practice that serves mostly private patients. This decision should be made on the basis of an objective evaluation and not an emotional response to the chaotic state of the current mental health care environment. For some practices in some markets, this is a viable option.

    This decision would mean that your practice can thrive without new sources of patients and without the backing of an alliance of other providers. It probably means that the market share for managed care is low or that you are already on one or more panels of providers. You will need to establish a marketing plan to be sure that you can continue to reach the private market you are now serving. And keep your eye on the market—it can change rapidly. Your plans need to include a method of monitoring the local environment so that you can anticipate changes that might weaken your patient base.

■   After assessing your situation, personal preferences, and the local market conditions, you may decide to build an informal alliance while continuing to practice alone or in a small group. This decision could help build your referrals and might provide you with new information about business practices. It will not help much in obtaining managed care or other contracts. If the managed care market share is low and your referral sources are strong, this can be a good plan.

Start collecting data on your performance record so that should you need to "prove" yourself to larger organizations, you will have the data to do so. Make sure that your business operations are running smoothly and efficiently so that your overhead expenses do not drive your rates higher than what others in the community are charging. Also, see the How to Form a Group section at the end of chapter 4, for the steps in putting together informal or formal groups.

■   After assessing your practice, personal preferences, and the local market conditions, you may decide to work toward joining or creating a much larger and more integrated affiliation of therapists. If the managed care market share is high, the competition for clients in your community is fierce, or if you need access to more sophisticated business management skills, this move can work well for you.

You have several avenues open to you in finding that larger affiliation.

• You can seek to join a large group practice already in existence. Collect the data on your treatment successes and costs and approach a group with whom you are compatible. (Also see the marketing section of chapter 6.)

• Look for other therapists who are interested in forming a new group practice either through merging present practices or by starting from scratch. Start out with discussions about what you want to create. Follow the steps in strategic planning listed later in this chapter to develop your mission and objectives. Make sure that the psychologists with whom you are meeting see not only the professional aspect of practice as you do but the business arrangements as well. When you have come to some agreement and the group has coalesced, contact a consultant or attorney to help you decide on the best model for the practice. (See the How to Form a Group section at the end of chapter 4.)

• If you are interested in forming a new organization such as an IPA or PPO rather than a new group practice, begin by stating your objectives clearly. Are you seeking to have greater influence in contracting? If so, you may want to find other practitioners who are interested in putting together an organization with this goal. If you also want to gain access to better business management, consider who might join you in a GWW or a management service contract. In any case, get expert help. Do not create a new organization just for the sake of having something new. If it will not serve to achieve your goals, do not consider it.

Of these options, not making any changes in your present practice—standing pat—will cost you little money. You may need to allocate a larger amount of your operating budget to marketing, but no cash outlay is required. Creating or joining an informal alliance will cost you more in time than in cash. However, working toward a larger, more integrated group can be expensive in both time and money. Move cautiously. Make sure that you are creating the right organization before committing more than sweat equity. Most new organizations require 12–18 months to move from conception to operation—a period in which money can be consumed rapidly by consultants, attorneys, and staff. (For more information on consultants, see chapter 6 and the Choosing and Using Consultants section at the end of this chapter.)

Other Options

For many psychologists, employment in a psychiatric hospital, public mental health agency, or private service provides them with an opportunity to conduct their professional lives without worrying about running a business. Many organizations offer full- or part-time employment for qualified therapists and counselors.

Another alternative that does not involve "general" practice is the development of a special expertise. Some examples might be practices that are limited to cases of traumatic stress disorders, working with hostages, or an aspect of forensics (psychological autopsy, expert witness in criminal cases). Specialists usually need not be concerned with standard fees but can charge according to the complexity of the case and the value of their expertise. Few therapists, however, have the opportunity to develop such expertise except as a part of their general practice, and many years of experience are required to rise to the status of expert.

Some psychologists, faced with an exceptionally competitive local market, have diversified their practices by combining therapy, part-time employment, cases requiring special expertise, teaching, or research. If you decide to develop aspects of your business other than traditional therapy, keep in mind that you will need separate marketing plans for each product or "line."

Planning

In the same way that good therapy is based on good treatment planning, you will need an action plan to begin or revitalize your practice. A good plan will help you determine what you need to do first. Plans are generally described in three levels: (a) strategic, the long-range plans for the enterprise; (b) operational, the medium-range objectives for reaching a defined goal; and (c) day-to-day activity plans.

Strategic Planning

Strategic planning in any organization defines or redefines the purpose of the organization, establishes policies that will guide the enterprise and states the long-range goals. Practice strategy is the pattern of decisions that

- Determines and clearly states the practice goals and establishes policies and plans for achieving them
- Defines the nature of the business or services
- Sets forth the economic and human principles that make up the organizational culture
- States the nature (economic and noneconomic) of the contribution it wants to make to its stakeholders (owners, employees, customers, the community, or society it serves).

Strategic planning differs from operational planning in that it is longer range, broader in scope, concerns changes and discontinuity in the environment, and requires visionary thinking.

Competitive practices do not just happen. They must be planned. The strategic planning process builds on the strengths of a practice, its principals, and their aspirations. It modifies the aspirations with information about the environment in which the practice operates. The discipline of establishing business objectives and defining and scheduling actions to accomplish them invigorates the day-to-day management process. Remember the old adage, "If you don't know where you are going, you can choose any road."

Without a vision of what you want your practice to be, it is difficult to make midcourse adjustments in response to changes in the environment. Responding to crises takes the time of managers and principals and keeps them from paying attention to growth and innovation. Pursuing only short-term goals is shortsighted and will lead to complacency. An active planning process sends signals throughout the practice or company—communicating the vision, reinforcing the culture, and empowering employees to act in the organization's interests as well as their own. The existence of objectives and action plans creates a foundation for specific actions and areas of responsibility.

The steps in planning are deceptively simple. You will find, however, that serious consideration of each step is challenging, requires time and effort, and, if others are involved, raises questions that must be resolved.

Step 1: *Write a mission statement.*

Describe your practice as you wish it to be 5 years from now. Consider the following:

- What business should we be in? What business are we in (basic purpose)?
- Who are our customers? (Consider all clients and purchasers of care.)
- What are our "products"? Are any of them unique?
- Do we serve or wish to serve a particular market sector?
- How do we deliver our services (form of practice, referral patterns)?

- How have our products or services changed in the past 3 years? How are they likely to change in the next 3 years?
- What are our economic concerns (high income per principal, maintenance of current levels of income, growth or expansion, holding on to market share)?
- Are there ideological issues that should be incorporated into the mission statement (quality, innovation, image, leadership, risk taking)?
- What special consideration do we have for the stakeholders in the practice (owners, officers, founders, parent organization, employees, shareholders)?

To develop your mission statement, review the Fact Sheet in the PATs.

Your mission statement need not carry a response to all of these questions, but each should be carefully considered, discussed among the principals or owners, and stated as clearly as possible. The mission statement is often called the "vision" of the business, and you will return to it many times as you make major decisions about the future of the practice.

Step 2: Conduct an external environmental analysis.

Look at the health care environment, the business economics in the community in which you practice, and the trends in the community that may affect the viability and growth of your practice. Consider the regulatory, political, economic, technological, social, and competitive forces that could affect you. How might the market for your services change? Is the basic structure of the health care industry being modified? Are the resources you need likely to be available when you need them? In conducting this analysis, review the text of chapter 2 and your responses to the Area Market Data, Referral Base, Patient–Payer Profile, and Business Management forms in the PATs.

Step 3: Check your practice's strengths and weaknesses.

What resources do you have for competing in the market? What deficiencies exist in your practice? List strengths and weaknesses in strategically important categories, such as:

- Services (existing and planned)
- Product or service quality
- Human resources
- Delivery capability
- Reputation in the community
- Financial status
- Office appearance and ambiance.

All of the forms in the PATs will help you delineate the best aspects of your practice and those elements that need improvement. Also, complete the Quality Improvement section of the PATs to catalog clients' responses to your practice.

Step 4: *Formulate the objectives of the practice.*

This step results in specific statements about what the practice wants to become at some point in the future. On the basis of the mission statement, the objectives should state what is to be accomplished and when the objectives should be completed. Keep the number of objectives small and phrase them carefully. Do not try to say how the objectives should be pursued; there may be many ways to accomplish the same end. Just try to state what the end results would be like.

Some typical objectives might be (a) to provide more than 50% of marriage counseling services in Whalen County by 1995; (b) to add a quality crisis intervention product to the services of the group by June 1994; (c) to develop an alliance with other providers that will increase referrals by 15% by August 1994; and (d) to increase the number of clients in managed care markets by 10% within 2 years.

Some guidelines for writing objectives[1] include the following:

- Start with the word *to*, followed by an action verb.
- Specify a single key result to be accomplished and a target date for its accomplishment.
- Wherever possible, state the maximum cost factors.
- Make it specific and quantitative so that its accomplishment can be measured and verified.
- Avoid the "why" and "how"; state only the "what" and "when."
- Each objective should relate directly to the mission statement.
- Each objective should be realistic, attainable, and easily understandable by those who will be expected to attain it.
- Objectives should be in writing and referred to periodically by the principals in the practice as well as other employees who are responsible for actions related to the objectives.

Operational Planning

Once the objectives have been established and agreed on, the plan moves from strategy to operations. The results of Steps 5 and 6 should be a list of activities designed to reach a specific goal, a schedule for completing each activity, and an assignment of responsibility.

Step 5: *Develop alternatives for accomplishing each objective and choose the best for implementation.*

You might consider the following process for completing this step:

- Assign the development of alternatives to one or more persons who will be involved in accomplishing the objective. Suggest that they brainstorm as many alternatives as possible for reaching the objective.

---

[1]Adapted from *Management by Objectives and Results* by George L. Morrisey. Addison-Wesley Publishing Co., Reading, MA.

- When they have exhausted ideas for new alternatives, ask the group to rank them according to the group's best estimate of their feasibility.
- Develop the first few on the ranked list by noting all of the human resources that will be necessary for accomplishment and project the labor costs. Estimate direct costs for equipment, materials, and so forth, related to the objective.
- Using the new data on cost, rerank all of the objectives by feasibility.
- Choose the alternative that emerges as the most feasible and plan for its implementation. Specify the separate tasks that must be completed, assign the responsibility for each task, and assign a target date.

When all of the objectives have been processed, prepare a list (with details) and arrange all of the objectives and tasks on a master schedule. This process often reveals that the human and financial resources needed for all objectives are excessive or poorly timed. Make adjustments as needed.

For solo practitioners or small partnerships, follow the same process even though you may be working alone. Friends and relatives can serve as a brainstorming group in some cases. The primary purpose of this step is to generate many ideas and activities that could accomplish your objectives.

Step 6: *Implement the tasks that will lead to the accomplishment of the objectives.*

When a task is assigned to an individual within the practice, make sure that he or she understands and accepts the responsibility and recognizes that an individual's performance rating will include an evaluation of how well the task was performed.

Monthly—no less than quarterly—evaluate the results of the activities. Have the activities produced the desired results? Is there new information that suggests that different alternatives should be chosen? Are tasks being completed on schedule? Make adjustments as needed.

Do not despair if there does not seem to be time to accomplish all the tasks you have set out for yourself. Alter your schedule and try again. The worst action you can take is to file the plan in a desk drawer until you can "get to it." At the end of the year, you'll be no closer to your ideal practice than you are today.

Strategic planning is never finished; operational planning usually follows an annual cycle. At least annually, the practice principals should reevaluate the progress made toward the overall objectives of the practice and determine whether the direction should remain unchanged. At the same time, the mission statement should be reviewed, the assessments of the external and internal climate should be updated, and new objectives added when appropriate. The cycle continues year after year and gets easier to complete each time.

6

Making Your Practice a Successful Business

Putting Business Into Practice and Practice Into Business

The previous chapters in this Guidebook clearly show that, to compete effectively for business, practices must be able to combine the psychologist's goal of providing empathic and astute responses to the client's personal needs with goal-directed, well-organized, modern business practices. These goals need not clash. Good business practices will support and maintain your ability to use good clinical skills. But remaining competitive will require fresh ideas, adoption of new "best practices" as they are identified, and continuous improvement of operations.

The knowledge and skills needed to run a successful business are attainable through reading, education, and working with experts. Individuals with expertise can review each of the systems needed to run your practice and suggest ways to maintain or improve them. It may be a good use of your time to seek help from others who have demonstrated business ability so that you can spend time doing what you do best: working with clients. Naturally, the cost of hiring outside expertise is greater than learning to do it yourself. Furthermore, if you rely on someone else's judgment and do not learn all of the options for yourself, you may give up some control. Of course, the "do-it-yourself" and "buy it" options can be mixed, allowing you to set up those business procedures with which you are comfortable and hiring someone to help you with others.

In some locations, a practice can purchase business office services from commercial companies. A business office service company may lease space for your practice, purchase or lease equipment, manage support staff, and operate billing and collection services. Alternatively, limited services may be available through contracts. For example, billing and insurance claims processing services exist in most metropolitan areas. For a fee (a percentage of the money involved, a flat fee per month, or a fee per form processed), these services will handle the accounts receivable for your practice. As always, the benefit may be offset by the loss of control over how one's business transactions are conducted.

This chapter contains suggestions and guidelines for the business aspects of your practice. Most of the suggestions are applicable to a wide range of psychological services businesses. Most will apply to one-person offices as well as to large clinics or group practice settings.

Business Systems

One way to view the operation of an office is to delineate the systems needed for its operation. Although some systems overlap, administration (scheduling, patient records, office space and ambiance, business insurance), finance (accounting, credit and collection), insurance claims filing, communications, personnel, computers and management information, quality improvement, and marketing are sufficiently discrete to warrant attention by the owners or principals in a practice.

How should you deal with these business systems? Where do you start? How can you ensure that your practice will operate the way you want? What are your responsibilities?

You can approach your business operation in three steps: Establish the policies that will govern the practice, specify the procedures that will fulfill the intent of the policies, and ensure that these procedures are carried out in daily practice.

1. Review the business systems listed in this chapter. For each, determine the policies you want your practice to follow. Answer such questions as

    • How do I want the telephone answered and by whom?
    • To what degree do I want the practice to be involved in filing insurance claims?
    • What will be the credit and collection policies of this practice?
    • How large a staff do I want? Do I want to be the employer or shall I seek other staffing arrangements?

    Cover all the systems thoroughly and consider any changes you would like to make in your present practice. Even if you operate your practice without any assistance, state your policies in writing. It is an exercise that will help you to think about your practice in a business sense and establish your personal responsibilities for each function.

2. Think about each of the policies that you have just developed. Describe the procedure that should be followed to make the policy come to life. This step is particularly important if others will be responsible for carrying out the procedures. If you already have a procedure manual, make sure that it is accurate, complete, and current.

    For example, suppose that you have decided to contract with a telephone answering service for after-hours calls and calls received while you are with a patient. Write out the instructions that you give to the answering service: the phrase that you want used when they answer the telephone, the information they are to provide to callers under various circumstances (after-hours, therapist busy, etc.), and how you plan to evaluate their service.

3. If you have others working for and with you, their performance standards and evaluations should state clearly which of the procedures are their responsibilities. When performance is reviewed, each staff member should be told how well he or she is performing each task. Make sure staff understand their accountability.

    If you choose to operate your practice alone, state how you will evaluate whether you have followed the procedures and carried out the policies as you intended. Conduct a quarterly evaluation—at the same time as a review of your financial condition—and make adjustments on the basis of your evaluation.

As you read the suggestions listed under each business system, keep three factors in mind: policies, procedures, and evaluation of performance.

Administrative Systems

Office Space and Ambiance

It may be redundant to say that the costs of operating a practice are increasing rapidly. Office space is more expensive; the decorating and upkeep expenses continue to rise. However, today's purchasers and clients expect therapists to have a conveniently located, attractive office in pleasant surroundings.

Many psychologists practice in informal settings in their homes or in small offices to promote a casual, inviting atmosphere—deliberately avoiding the look of a medical institution or a bustling business office. Often, the office space is small and intimate, business arrangements are individualized for clients, and policies and procedures are flexible. Although this design may reduce stress for clients and provide an amicable setting for therapy, the relaxed atmosphere may adversely affect important business operations, resulting in inappropriate and inefficient practices. The small, intimate setting may be seen by others as meager or scanty, the personalized service erratic or inconsistent, and the flexible arrangements careless or haphazard. Financial policies and procedures designed for individual clients may deteriorate into poor collection procedures that affect the financial viability of the practice. The following suggestions are based on the experience of other mental health care providers.

- Select office space that represents the image you want for your practice. A homelike office is appropriate if you usually see one client at a time, need to demonstrate the security of the encounter, and wish to project a quiet, relaxed atmosphere. In some urban areas there may be little choice but to open an office in a high-rise. Although this is perhaps appropriate for a practice that provides testing and career counseling services, it presents more of a challenge to the provider interested in projecting a soothing, warm atmosphere. Review the long-range plans for your practice and try to describe the setting that would allow your plans to come to fruition.

- Choose a location for your practice that is easily accessible to your clients. Is the practice on public transportation lines? Are there safe, well-lit parking areas nearby? Is your office in a neighborhood that is convenient to your clients' residences or convenient to their places of employment? Knowing where your clients come from when they have appointments will help you to decide where to locate your office and what hours would be convenient for your clients' schedules.

- Investigate the feasibility of opening a satellite office so that you will be available in more than one location. You could share (or switch) offices with other psychologists who would like to have more than one location without significantly increasing your overhead expenses. Plan very carefully before opening two offices by yourself. The overhead created by maintaining two offices could be excessive, especially if your schedule is not filled at either location.

- Be sure that your office building has good access for disabled patients or those using wheelchairs. Elderly patients may also require special attention. The chairs in the reception area should have seats high enough for patients to sit comfortably and rise easily. Also, check the standards developed for the Americans With Disabilities Act to make sure your office and the building in which it is located conform to those standards.

- Make your reception area warm, approachable, and pleasant. Choose comfortable seating, good lighting, and decor that indicates an understanding of how light, color, texture and noise affect human emotions. Provide reading materials, such as general interest periodicals, to help clients relax while waiting. Some therapists have equipped their waiting rooms with sound-masking machines to ensure that therapy conducted nearby is not overheard.

- Ensure privacy and confidentiality in the office and consultation space. One possibility is to provide an exit that does not require the client to walk through the reception area when the client is leaving. Arrange the space and furniture so that when the receptionist is talking with others on the phone, the conversation cannot be heard in the reception area.

- Because it may be difficult for you to assess the office area from a visitor's perspective, ask a friend or family member who can be objective to visit your office and give you a "client's" evaluation. What are their impressions of the atmosphere? Is the area well maintained? Is privacy ensured? Does the space have both the ambiance that you want and a businesslike, professional image?

Scheduling

In today's competitive market, new clients calling for an appointment are seeking more than just a slot on your regular appointment schedule. They want a quick response to their need for a first appointment, convenient hours, an easy-to-find location, and compassionate handling of their requests. If any of these elements is missing, clients will call another therapist. You must consider carefully your new clients' first impressions. Here are some basic tips for your initial contact procedure that experienced practitioners know well:

- Establish the most client-pleasing method for answering your telephones because your first and continuing contact with your clients is often by telephone. Most clients would rather speak to a person than a machine, but you may need to have a service that provides both.

    If you generally answer your own phone, you will need a device to answer the phone when you are with a patient. During business hours, an answering machine with a gentle message asking the caller to leave a message or to call back at a time when you know you will be available should be sufficient. An answering service whose operators respond after a specified number of rings would be better. In either instance, you should be as definite as possible about when you will return the call. For example, asking the caller, "please leave a message and I will return the call within the hour" or "please leave a message and I will return the call between 11:00 and 11:30" is very reassuring to an anxious patient. In dealing with the answering service, indicate to them the time of day that you will return your calls so that they can convey that information to your callers. Be sure you make your return calls at the appointed time and, if the call concerns the patient's therapy, record the nature of the conversation in your patient records.

- If you use a telephone answering machine, the message should be changed for calls that you receive after-hours. Specify what the patient should do in an emergency or where you can be reached if the situation is urgent. Many practices use an answering machine during office hours and a service for after-hours calls.

- Purchase an appointment book or appointment software for your computer system. Determine the hours that you will see clients and block off the amount of time you want for each client. Some practitioners block more time for the initial appointment than for subsequent ones so that there is ample time to follow a standardized intake procedure and spend time with the patient. Others make the first appointment shorter—just enough time for you and the patient to determine whether you wish to continue working together. If you work with groups and families, you may want to block more time for them than for individual patients.

    If you work with other therapists in the same practice, there is no need to standardize your schedules. Your receptionist (and the computer software) can easily adapt to different hours for each therapist, different ways of handling new clients, and varying the length of appointments.

- Make sure that your practice maintains a schedule that is appropriate for the population you serve. If most of your clients are employed, you may need to establish some late afternoon, early morning, evening, or weekend hours to accommodate them.

- Set up your schedule so that clients who are on time for their appointments do not have to wait. If you find that you are always running late, block more time for each appointment or make it clear to your clients that you will be firm about starting and ending appointments on time.

- When you are building your practice, leave space in the schedule so that you can accommodate new clients immediately. New clients do not yet have a relationship with you or your practice, and a long wait to get on your schedule may cause them to seek care elsewhere. Simply leave some time everyday or every other day for new clients. If you do not fill those slots with a new client, use the time for personal marketing activities.

- Let your patients know your policy on canceling appointments. Many therapists ask their patients to give them at least 24 hours notice if they need to cancel an appointment. In some cases, you may wish to charge for a missed or canceled appointment. This should be clearly stated—in advance—to your clients.

Patient Records

Practitioners vary in the amount of detail they record and store in patient records. There are, however, some data that are essential for billing, insurance, and treatment (the clinical record). Often, authorization for release of information, consent to treatment, and payment agreement forms are also maintained in patient records. The APA's "Record Keeping Guidelines" in the Appendix of this Guidebook provides additional guidance on issues of record content, construction and control, retention, and disclosure.

Billing and insurance data. To maintain good business records, the following forms should be completed by clients and retained as part of their financial records. For reasons of confidentiality and convenience, these records should be kept separate from the clinical record. They will be used primarily by those responsible for billing procedures and filing insurance claims.

- At the time of the initial visit, ask your client to complete a form that contains all of the personal information that you might need to contact that client in the future and to bill for services or file insurance claims. A Sample Patient Information Sheet is provided at the end of this chapter.
- Establish a routine to update personal information if you are seeing a patient over a long period of time. Address, phone number, employment, marital status, and insurance carrier and coverage should be checked every 6 months to ensure that the information is current. For a Medicaid patient, maintain a current photocopy of his or her eligibility card because verification of eligibility on the date of service is required for Medicaid reimbursement.
- If most of your clients have insurance coverage for all or part of their treatment costs, you may want them to sign an authorization for release of information and records to third-party payers or utilization reviewers and an assignment of benefits statement. (An assignment of benefits permits you to file an insurance claim on behalf of your patient and receive the insurance reimbursement directly. Without assignment, the insurance company will pay the patient and you collect fees from the patient.) Sample forms for authorization for release of information and records, assignment, and Medicare consultation release are shown at the end of this chapter.
- Many practitioners ask their clients to read and sign a payment agreement indicating their willingness to assume financial responsibility for their treatment. However, it is important to carefully read any contracts you may have with MCOs concerning patients' financial responsibility; some MCOs do not permit providers to collect the remainder of their fee from the patient or to see the patient if the MCO has denied authorization for further treatment. This procedure often provides an opening to discuss arrangements for partial payments for those individuals who are unable to pay in full at the time of service. A sample Payment Agreement Form is shown at the end of this chapter.
- For your convenience, you may want to complete an Insurance Verification Form on each client. Such forms are particularly useful if you plan to file claims on behalf of your clients. Obtain from your clients or, with their permission, from their insurance company, a copy of their insurance plan or the handbook that describes their benefits. Record all of the information that might be useful in completing the insurance forms: identification of the policy and policyholder, appropriate group numbers, types and amount of coverage, extent of deductibles

and co-payments that will be the responsibility of the patient, precertification agreements, and so on. (A sample Insurance Verification form is shown at the end of this chapter.)

Clinical records. The record of a patient's treatment and progress has been almost exclusively for the therapist's review to aid in the treatment of that patient, to provide guidelines for treating other patients, and to document treatment should questions arise in the future. As mental health treatment comes under increasing scrutiny by insurance companies and MCOs, having good patient records takes on added importance. When you accept payment from third parties, you are often required to accept an audit of your records. The sensitive information contained in patient records is often sought by third parties, sometimes inappropriately. You will need to retain copies of consent forms allowing you to release such information. Parts of the "clinical" record become, in effect, a business record as well.

A thorough clinical record should include intake information, results of tests administered, progress notes, treatment plans, documentation of crisis therapy, termination summary, clinical analyses, and records of when and if treatment was approved by a third party. While some of this information can be legitimately requested by third party reviewers, other parts are strictly confidential. In cases were it is appropriate to release some part of this record, the therapist and not an outside auditor should be the one to go through the file and extract the necessary information. This ensures the client's confidentiality.

■ The organization of each record should follow a pattern. A logical organization might be as follows:

- intake information sheet
- statement of presenting problem or situation and history
- test results (if any)
- treatment plan
- medication record (if needed)
- progress notes (session summaries)
- consultation notes if patient is referred for additional care
- legal documents (release forms)
- termination summary with notes on aftercare and follow-up
- verification of contacts with third parties (precertifications, treatment plan extensions).

■ To ensure that the "business" portion of your records will stand up to questioning or examination by third parties, a review of your records should be conducted regularly. Sloppy documentation and record keeping may cause chart reviewers and claims adjustors to doubt the competence or integrity of the provider. To avoid problems later, conduct internal audits so that you will know how well you are doing, or have a trusted staff member help you with the review. Pull several active or recently closed records at random and see whether the following items are in the record, organized in a logical fashion, complete, legible, and understandable.

- Financial: For each visit indicated in the clinical record, is there a corresponding charge in the patient's payment record or insurance file? If you did not charge the client, is that also indicated in the records? Financial auditors are very suspicious when they cannot track each visit and its attendant charges.
- Treatment: Is a copy of the treatment plan in the record with goals, treatment methods, and means for assessing progress clearly described? If releasing this record would breach your client's confidentiality, do you have an appropriately distilled version? Do the progress notes relate specifically to the treatment plan without breaching confidentiality? Is the record free of jargon that might cause misinterpretation?
- Crisis management: If there is indication of any crisis during the patient's treatment period, is it properly documented? Has a standard procedure for evaluating suicide or homicide risk been used? Is a copy of the procedure included? Are potentially difficult or controversial clinical judgments fully discussed?

- Keep in touch with the medical reviewers of the insurance carriers with whom you work. Learn about their review procedures, anticipate what issues they face, anticipate the information they will need, and develop a rapport with them. When questions arise or an audit is scheduled, the good relationships that you and your staff have developed may make the audit process easier.
- Be sure you sign and date all entries and notations in the record. Sign all documents that are entered into the record.
- Be sure that your records are stored in a safe area and that access to the records is strictly limited. The major reason for creating a separate business file on each client is to reduce the need for another staff member (claims administrator or billing clerk) to see the file. Locked, fireproof file cabinets usually provide sufficient security. If your clinical records are computerized, be sure that access is limited by strictly controlled and frequently changed passwords and that a backup record is maintained in a safe place off-site.
- In the absence of specific state laws stating otherwise, the full clinical record on each patient should be maintained for at least 3 years after termination. A summary (or the full record) should be maintained for an additional 12 years before disposal. These guidelines are suggested by the APA's "Record Keeping Guidelines" (see the Appendix) and most professional liability insurers; check with your carrier for their recommendations. If you wish to summarize your records, schedule a time to do so every 6 months or at year's end.
- Establish a procedure for releasing records when required to do so. Check your state's laws for specific requirements because special rules usually apply to mental health records. (See the sample authorization for release of information and records at the end of this chapter.) *Never* release the original record; when required to supply a record, send a photocopy. Check with your attorney and professional liability insurance carrier whenever you have questions about record releases.
- If an insurance carrier or managed care company notifies you of an audit,

- Check your contract to determine whether you have agreed to such audits and review the procedures.
- Examine the identification of on-site auditors; make sure that the information you provide to off-site audits cannot jeopardize your patient's confidentiality.
- Make no changes in your records in anticipation of an audit. Alterations to your records will harm you far more than the original documentation (or lack of it).
- If in doubt about any aspect of the audit, contact your attorney. Make sure that you have all of the patient consent forms that are required by the laws in your state.
- If the audit agency or MCO claims that it has the patient's permission to look at his or her records, request a copy of the form.

Remember that your duty to protect the confidentiality of your patients is one of your primary concerns as a psychologist. Moreover, client–therapist communication is considered privileged and is therefore subject to certain legal protections. Make sure you have a clear sense of what information can be appropriately released and what information cannot.

Business insurance considerations

A good insurance program is an essential component of establishing a sound private practice in psychology. A well-designed insurance policy can contribute to the success of the practice by reducing some of the uncertainties psychologists face. Insurance is designed to protect you against losses. However, because it is not financially feasible to insure yourself against every possible loss, you should be prepared to absorb the small ones and make sure that you have the potentially large losses covered.

- Professional liability is designed to cover claims and legal actions that stem from alleged malpractice by a mental health services provider. Without professional liability, a therapist might be personally obligated to pay damages, attorney's fees, court costs, and other related expenses if a suit is decided in favor of a plaintiff. Even when a therapist is not found to have been negligent and is absolved in a malpractice action, the costs incidental to investigation and defense, coupled with the loss of earnings from time away from the practice, can be considerable.
- The amount of professional liability insurance you should carry will vary, depending on your type of practice, your specialty, the services that you will be providing, and the area in which you practice. If you serve on a panel for an MCO, be sure that you carry the amount of professional liability required by the contract.
- As an owner or lessor of property, you may be held legally responsible for an accident or mishap occurring on the premises that is attributable to your neglect. Although the incidence of such accidents is relatively low, check with your insurance agent to see what level of coverage is recommended in your area.
- If your practice provides an automobile or if you use your personal automobile

in your work, be sure that the automobile liability insurance includes bodily injury coverage and property damage liability. Also, check whether you need insurance to cover employees who might be injured while performing a service related to your practice.

■ Workers' Compensation insurance covers employees' illnesses and accidents that are related to work. State law determines how workers' compensation plans are funded; frequently, all employers are required to pay into a state fund set aside for this purpose. Check with your agent to determine the requirements.

■ Depending on the location and ownership of your office space, you may need fire, burglary, theft, and comprehensive damage insurance. The value of furniture and equipment should be included in the policy.

■ Fidelity bonds (bonding insurance) can be purchased to cover all employees who handle the funds of the practice. It allows recovery of some losses in case of embezzlement.

■ Health insurance for principals, employees, and their families is a valued benefit. Small businesses (fewer than 10 employees) in today's market have difficulty obtaining group health insurance at reasonable rates. If group insurance is not available, obtain a personal policy to cover you and your family even though this may not be a deductible business expense. Some states have special insurance laws for small employers. Check with your insurance agent to see if this is an option for you.

■ Disability insurance is designed to replace a portion of your earned income in the event of a disability caused by an accident or illness. It is imperative that the principals in the practice be adequately covered. The funds paid to you if you are disabled are often taxable as personal income.

■ Related to disability insurance is office overhead insurance. When a therapist is incapacitated, the office overhead continues. Overhead insurance assumes part or all of the cost of maintaining an office and staff during your period of disability.

For tax purposes, you can deduct from your business income the cost of insurance that protects you against professional liability losses, fire and casualty losses of office equipment and supplies, and office overhead insurance. Other insurance may not be deductible under Internal Revenue Service regulations. Check with your tax advisor, accountant, or attorney to determine under what conditions these insurance premiums can be considered deductible. And keep your eye on the market. A wide variety of insurance products are available in the market, and they are being constantly redesigned.

Financial Practices

In some markets, therapists have operated their practices on a "cash and carry" basis. Clients understood that they were expected to pay for services either before service, at the time of service, or at the end of each month in which services were provided. If bills were produced, they were handwritten. Therapists may or may not have provided the information needed by clients to file claims with their insurance companies. Clients may have been reluctant to file claims anyway. Thus, the practice could avoid establishing elaborate payment policies, billing procedures, or collection policies.

It is increasingly difficult, however, to find clients who are willing to assume the full cost of treatment without support from insurance. If you treat patients in an inpatient facility, you must prepare a bill or depend on someone who does. Medicare and Medicaid regulations require that you bill the patients covered by those programs and file claims for them. If you see clients who are unable to pay in full at time of service but are willing to arrange for smaller, longer term payments, it will be necessary to prepare bills that reflect those arrangements. And all MCOs require that they be "billed" for services even when you are being reimbursed on a capitation basis.

Payment options are rapidly changing from traditional fee for service to discounted fees, relative value scales, capitation, weighted value, and medicare-type rate systems. Most practices have an ever-shifting mix of these payment systems to track; financial data management becomes an important function. The following are a few financial tips:

- Establish the payment policies that you plan to follow in your practice. Be sure that each member of your office staff understands the procedures he or she is to follow in order to enact the policies. Ask your staff (or check the books yourself) at the end of each week to determine whether most payments are being collected as planned. If not, correct the situation.
- Determine your overhead rate. Overhead is the amount you spend on all business expenses (e.g., rent or mortgage, staff salaries and benefits, office equipment and supplies, etc.). If you are the principal in the practice, your salary or draw from the practice is usually not included. The overhead rate is determined by dividing the amount of business expense by gross income. It is difficult to state what is a "good" overhead rate because the nature of mental health practices varies greatly. It is probably more important to track the rate on a monthly basis so that inflationary trends are noted quickly. Whatever the rate, a prudent business owner occasionally checks each item to determine whether the cost is necessary and reasonable.
- Develop a system for determining the cost of delivering a service by type of service. Specifically, calculate the fixed expenses, variable expenses, and professional service fee required for each product of the practice. Using these basic figures, you can determine approximately how much it actually costs you to provide an hour of service or an average for all the services for a given diagnosis. This information is crucial for dealing with contracts with managed care arrangements or insurance carriers that seek discounted fees. Does the fee arrangement that they offer cover your costs and provide a profit?
- Determine the payer mix of your practice income by calculating the percentage each category of payer contributed to total gross receipts. Most practices cannot afford to rely too heavily on a single carrier or purchaser of care. Should your relationship with that purchaser change, the financial impact on your practice could be disastrous. Keeping track of how many patients come from each payer source, and the receipts for their treatment will give you a picture of your

income flow. You will know if the payer mix shifts in ways that are harmful to your income, and you can adapt your marketing to accommodate for the shift.

■ Working with your accountant, you can establish financial management systems that will help you calculate the effect of new contracts to deliver services. By loading into the system the fees offered in the contract, the number of new clients anticipated, and the additional administrative costs of contract compliance, you can determine how the new income will affect your income if all other portions of your practice remain constant.

■ Track financial data that will help you market your services. Today's market requires that psychologists must compete with each other on both the effectiveness of service and cost. MCOs and other purchasers of care collect financial data on their providers and compare one with another. Therapists who are not cost-effective may be dropped from the provider panel. Establish your own tracking system that will give you data to compare with those obtained by the carriers and serve as an early warning system that your services are becoming less cost-effective.

■ If you contract with any third-party payer to provide services at a rate lower than your regular fee (either by discount or acceptance of the third party's fee schedule), you may want your accounting system to track the difference between what you would charge if you were treating a direct-pay client and what the third party pays. This system allows you to track how much (in theory) you have actually given up by working through a third party. Your accountant can help you to set up the procedures for recording both actual charges and negotiated or contracted charges.

Billing, Credit, and Collection

The policies that a practice establishes about payment, billing, and collection are inextricably linked to how you choose to handle insurance claims filing. Will you file claims for all clients or will you provide them with information that will permit them to file their own claims? Will you require payment of deductibles and co-payments at the time of service or bill clients for their portion of the bill only after the insurance company has paid its portion? Working with third-party payers increases the costs of the practice: the cost of bookkeeping and billing functions, the delay in cash flow while waiting for a third party to pay, the need to establish collections procedures, and the reduction in income resulting from the discounts required by many third-party payers. However, in most markets, it is difficult to operate a financially sound practice without third-party involvement.

Assuming that your practice performs its own bookkeeping and collection procedures, here are some practical suggestions to help you. Your headaches will be fewer if you decide to computerize the financial aspect of your practice (accounts payable and receivable, payroll, collections). If you choose not to computerize initially, purchase business forms from vendors that will help organize your accounting. Regardless of whether your system is manual or computer, here are some tips to make things easier:

- Explain fees, billing, and collection practices to your clients. Develop a client information handout that tells clients how to make or change appointments (to avoid a no-show charge), how insurance claims will be handled, your billing procedures, and all other business arrangements important to the client and to your practice. The handout may be a brochure or a few pages on your letterhead. Make it easy for your clients to learn about your business procedures. (See the Client Information Brochure instructions at the end of this chapter.)

- Let clients know what forms of payment you will accept (in addition to insurance coverage, if that is your choice). Cash, checks, and credit cards are generally accepted forms of payment in most larger practices. Contact your bank for credit card arrangements and fees.

- Most practices seek at least partial payment at the time of service. This is a good business practice and may, in some cases, provide a form of discipline for your patients. If patients indicate they are not able to pay in full at the time of their appointments, you can work out a schedule for partial payments. Remember that your overhead costs are increased every time you prepare and mail a bill. Work out office procedures that minimize the number of times you bill a patient for the same debt.

- When your clients arrive for their first appointment or before, ask them to complete a client information form (see the Patient Records section). Be sure to ask for information that will help in locating the client if collection procedures are necessary. Complete insurance information should be provided on that form and, if you plan to submit insurance claims for your patients, be sure that you ask them to assign their insurance payments to you in return. Without a statement signed by your patient authorizing payment of fees directly to you, all payments from the insurance company will be sent to the patient and you will have to collect the entire debt from your patient. If you are filing claims for your patients, they should be asked to assign their benefits. (See the sample Payment Agreement and Authorization for Assignment of Benefits forms at the end of this chapter.)

- Bills for unpaid balances should be sent to your clients promptly and regularly. The first bill—assuming that you are not pursuing a full-payment-at-time-of-service policy—should be mailed within 2 weeks of the date of service. Subsequent bills might be scheduled every 30 days thereafter.

  If a patient is not paying his or her bills, you or your office staff should discuss the situation with the patient as soon as nonpayment is obvious. This may be "grist" for the therapeutic mill. Make a schedule for partial payments if that is mutually agreeable.

- Consider turning over bad debts to a collection agency when your attempts to collect unpaid bills have failed. The agency—for a fee of 20%–40% of what they collect—will make further attempts to obtain payment. Small bills may not be worth pursuing; write them off your books as uncollectible. Collection agencies often are linked to a credit bureau and are in a position to affect a client's credit rating. Be sure you select an agency experienced in collecting psychologists' accounts or those of other health professionals. Such agencies are more likely to handle your clients with understanding, patience, gentle firmness, and attention to necessary confidentiality and privacy. This limits your exposure to the risk of an expensive lawsuit.

Financial Management

Good financial management is essential to good private practice. If you ignore the rudimentary financial principles, you will soon find yourself short of cash and in trouble with the Internal Revenue Service (IRS). Develop a sound system for handling the income and expenses from your practice.

Your accounting system, whether manual or computerized, should provide

- a daily listing of all clients and the charges for services to them (or an indication of "no charge")
- a daily listing of receipts (cash, checks, or credit card charges)
- a daily balance
- a daily update of accounts receivable
- a complete record of deposits and other bank transactions
- an individual record for each patient showing charges and payments.

Furthermore, the system should aggregate similar kinds of expenses and payments. For example, at month's end, the system should provide an income and expense statement for that month and year to date. Generally, all income is lumped together as professional income, but you may want a breakdown of income by payer (private insurance, managed care contracts, direct pay, etc.). Expenses should be categorized by type: rent, insurance, supplies, staff salaries and benefits, and so on. Your accountant can help you to set up an effective manual bookkeeping system or select a software accounting package for your computer.

- If there are several therapists in the practice, you will, of course, have a business checking account for all business transactions. Even if you are practicing alone, it is imperative that you establish a business bank account to make sure that you keep business funds separate from personal funds.

  A few banks offer checking and high-yield interest (money market) in the same business account. If your bank does not offer such a service, consider putting all receipts into a high-yield account and then transfer to a checking account enough money at bill-paying time to cover all of the outstanding bills. In this way, your receipts are earning money for most of the month. Make sure that the high-yield account allows you to transfer money into your checking account without a substantial penalty for early withdrawal.
- Receipts should be deposited daily. Establish a routine for endorsing the checks that you receive (get a "For Deposit Only" stamp), and gather the cash received for a daily trip to the bank or a night deposit.
- If clients frequently pay in cash, establish a secure place to store the cash. Be sure that the money in the cash drawer balances at the end of the day.
- Your bank can help you determine whether accepting credit card charges for bills is appropriate for your practice and can help you obtain that service. Remember that the credit card company—not your practice—will be respon-

sible for collecting all the items that have been charged on their card. Accepting credit cards can reduce your collection costs.

- When you begin your practice or form a partnership or corporation, request from your local IRS office Form SS-4, Application for Employer Identification Number. You will have an employer identification number assigned to you so that the taxes you pay will be properly credited to your practice. In most states, this request will trigger contact by the state taxing authority. Ask for a copy of *Tax Guide for Small Businesses*, Publication 334, and *Your Federal Income Tax*, Publication 17, to learn more about your tax responsibilities (also review the information on how various practice forms are taxed in chapter 4).

- You are required by law to keep records that will enable you to prepare a complete and accurate income tax return. Although the law does not require any special record format, you must retain all receipts, canceled checks, and other evidence to prove amounts claimed as business deductions. The tax guides just listed will be helpful to you in determining what are legitimate business expenses.

  Source records for the income or deductions that appear on a return must be kept until the statute of limitations expires. Usually, this is 3 years from the date the return was due or filed or 2 years from the date paid, whichever occurs later. Copies of your tax returns should be kept and may be helpful in preparing future returns.

Financial Checkup

A financial checkup on your business can help you to determine whether you are operating effectively. Your accountant can assist you with the checkup because most of the critical information can be pulled directly from your bookkeeping system: profit and loss statement, accounts receivable aging records, and insurance claim files.

Here are five easy steps for your checkup:

- Start with an overview of the practice. Calculate the total charges for each of the past 3 years, compare them with total receipts for the same periods, and determine the collection ratio. The collection ratio is total charges minus foreseen adjustments divided by total receipts. Comparative data for mental health practices are not available, but if your collection ratio is lower than 85%, consider becoming more aggressive in your billing and collection practices. No matter what the ratio is, concentrate on ways to make it higher.

- Review your accounts receivable. Use the monthly average for each of the 3 years or select a month and use the actual amount outstanding at that month in each of the 3 years. An acceptable level of accounts receivable would be between 15% and 20% of total receipts. Again, no matter what the level is, try to improve it.

- Determine your practice costs (overhead). Total overhead includes the fixed and variable costs of doing business: payroll, office space, malpractice and other insurance premiums, supplies, depreciation on equipment and furniture, continuing education, and all other tax-deductible costs. Divide your receipts by overhead expenses to determine the percentage of total receipts. Overhead expenses for therapists generally run between 25% and 35% of annual receipts but can vary greatly on the basis of the services of the practice.

■ Calculate the amount of charges written off to professional courtesy, write-offs (charity, bad debts, etc.), agreed-on discounts, and refunds. Divide the total charges by the amount written off to determine the adjustment rate. Be sure the rate is low enough that the financial viability of your practice is not threatened.

■ Compute net income before taxes. The net income includes all of your compensation (salary, bonuses, dividends, etc.) and profit.

What changes do the figures for the past 3 years indicate? Are there any positive trends (income rising, overhead decreasing as a percentage of charges, decreasing accounts receivable)? Any negative trends? If the overhead has changed significantly, was it planned (additional staff, new lease, change in benefits)? Or was it due to reduced revenues? Are you writing off more to bad debt? Check your billing and collection policies. Are you writing off more to contracts with discounted fee schedules? Are the discounted fees covering your costs? Although you might not change your financial management plans on the basis of the answer to any one question in this list, you can get an overall financial picture of your practice and some ideas for where to look for improvements.

Insurance Claim Processing

As indicated in the Financial Management section, the financial policies of a practice are inextricably linked to your decisions about insurance and managed care contracts and therefore cannot be ignored. In many practices, payments from third-party payers represent as much as 75% of the practice income. The following are some suggestions for determining how to deal with third parties and how to help your clients understand their financial responsibilities when a third party is involved.

First, here is an explanation of some insurance terms:

■ **Assignment or assignment of benefits:** Assignment is the authorization by the insured (client) for the insurer (insurance company or MCO) to pay benefits directly to the provider (you). If a patient does not assign benefits, you cannot receive payment directly from the insurance company, and you must collect all charges from the patient. In some insurance programs, accepting assignment may impose additional regulations and claims filing procedures. Read your contracts carefully to make sure there are no strings attached.

■ **Coding:** A variety of numerical and alpha-numeric codes are used to report the patient's diagnosis and the procedures and services performed by a caregiver. The use of numbers to represent complex procedures facilitates communication between providers and claims payers. The three most frequently used coding systems are listed below.

- **Current Procedure Terminology (CPT) codes:** The CPT is a systematic listing and numerical coding of procedures and services of health care providers. The codes in CPT are maintained by the American Medical Association. A five-digit code for each service provided (individual psychotherapy, group or family psychotherapy, etc.) is reported on the insurance claim form along with the charges for each.
- **Revised third edition and fourth edition of the *Diagnostic and Statistical Manual of Mental Disorders (DSM)* codes:** The *DSM* is psychiatric diagnostic typology developed by the American Psychiatric Association and used for reporting diagnoses on most insurance claims. Diagnostic codes indicate the necessity for the treatment provided.
- *International Classification of Disease–Ninth Revision–Clinical Modification codes:* These diagnostic codes are required in many states for Medicare and Medicaid claims. Some states also accept *DSM* codes. They are maintained by the World Health Organization.

- **Claim forms:** Nearly all insurance carriers accept the HCFA's claim form 1500 for filing claims. Medicare and some Medicaid programs require that service providers submit the HCFA 1500 for their patients who are in those programs.
- Each practice should establish a policy regarding insurance filing. You can be guided on your policy selection by reviewing the number of patients who are covered by insurance and by local custom. If most therapists file claims for their clients, you will want to do so too. Some of the choices are the following:

  - Accept all insurance coverage, accept assignment, and bill the insurance company for services and wait for the payment before billing the patient for the balance that was not paid by insurance. Your patients will appreciate your filing insurance claims on their behalf. However, the practice forgoes income from the service rendered for several weeks while the insurance claim is being processed. Furthermore, in some cases, agreeing to participate in an insurance program limits the amount that the practitioner can charge.
  - Accept all insurance coverage, accept assignment, and request payment for the patient's co-payment or deductible at the time of service; bill the insurance company on behalf of the patient. Getting some payment at the time of service helps the cash flow of the practice. This policy requires a careful examination of the insurance coverage of each patient to determine the amount of co-payment or deductible for collection at time of service.
  - Request payment in full from the patient at time of service; provide all of the information necessary for the patient to file a claim with his or her insurance company. This choice may seem harsh, particularly for patients who need to spread payments over time. It does, however, bring payment into the practice more quickly than the other options.
  - Collect nothing at the time of service; bill the patient on a regular basis for the unpaid balance of his or her bill. This option puts the practice at financial risk for all collections, increases overhead costs by requiring the production and mailing of regular statements, and delays payment for services provided.

This plan may be fine for long-term patients with whom you have established satisfactory payment schedules.

Do not forget that the practice *must* complete and submit all bills that are to be paid by Medicare. The patient is not permitted to file his or her own claims. In some states, the same requirement may apply to Medicaid patients.

- If you plan to file claims for any of your clients, establish a routine to gather the information necessary to complete the insurance form, prepare the form promptly, and forward it to the insurance company. Depending on your schedule of visits with your client, you may wish to file a claim immediately after each visit or for all the visits during 1 month.
- Decide when to resubmit insurance claims that you believe are underpaid by the insurance company. State clearly the reason for the resubmission and request a second review. If the claim is not paid after resubmission, consider appealing the case. A claim that is only for a small amount or for unusual treatment or circumstances may not be worth the time and effort of an appeal. A large, unpaid claim or a slight underpayment of a frequently occurring claim can be worth an appeal. Most insurance carriers have an appeal process that appears in the contract you sign. If you do have not have a contract, call the company's claims office and ask for a copy of the appeal process.
- Whether you file claims for your clients or simply provide them with the data for filing on their own, you need to become familiar with the diagnostic and procedure codes used for claim processing. Proper coding speeds the payment process.
- When a client is divorced or a child of divorced or separated parents, the insurance problems can become complicated. These are some of the situations that arise:

  - Because of the divorce, the client may no longer be covered by his or her ex-spouse's insurance and has no personal insurance. Treat the patient as a private patient and request some payment at time of service.
  - The noncustodial parent is required by the divorce decree to pay for insurance and medical expenses for the child. If you choose to accept insurance payment through the noncustodial parent, insist on assignment of benefits and be sure you obtain all of the information required to send the bill.
  - The child is from a blended family whose insurance covers some family members but not all and it is not obvious whether your client is covered. Treat the patient as a private patient. In anticipation of collection problems, some practices require that the parent or guardian who brings a minor child take responsibility for payment of treatment fees. The practice provides all of the data necessary for the parent or guardian to file for insurance, obtain reimbursement from the ex-spouse, or both.

Regardless of how these situations are handled, it is in the best interests of the practice to find out as much as possible about any insurance that might provide coverage. If necessary, get your client's permission and then call his or her employer (the purchaser of the insurance) to determine whether your client is covered. With this information, you and your client can agree on a treatment plan that fits the circumstances.

Communications

Telephone communications, covered in the Scheduling section, is so important to the efficient operation of a practice that some points are worth repeating.

- Establish your telephone answering policies after careful thought about the needs of your clients and efficient use of your time.
- Be sure that whatever answering device or service you use is "tuned in" to your practice. Be clear about when you will return calls and how clients can reach you in emergencies.
- Voice mail systems that permit callers to leave messages may be more convenient for your clients. Some systems allow the caller to override the message system if help is needed immediately. By pressing a stated number, the caller can be transferred to a secretary or receptionist or to another phone that signals a need for your personal response.
- Whatever system you choose, check occasionally to ensure that the system operates as you designed it or, in the case of answering services, that the calls are being answered as you have instructed the service. Just call your own number and listen carefully, as if you were your own client.
- If you are just starting your practice, be wary of buying too little or too much equipment. There is virtually no market for used telephone equipment, so if you should find that your purchase is inadequate for the size of your practice, you generally have to purchase all new equipment. Think about how you plan to use the telephones, make a list of the number of phone lines, extensions, and peripheral equipment (intercom, speed dial, etc.) that you need, and then shop around before buying.

In today's high-tech world, additional communications equipment can make the practice operate more smoothly. Although most therapists' offices are not equipment heavy, there are some labor-saving devices that should be considered.

- A fax machine can reduce the amount of time needed to send documents to third-party payers or to other professionals. You may include an electronic device in your computer that can send and receive a fax or you can purchase a separate fax machine. It is important to ensure the confidentiality of information transmitted by fax.
- If you deal with clients who need immediate access to you or if you work with patients in a number of hospitals or institutions, consider leasing or buying a cellular phone, mobile phone, or paging (beeper) system. The lease or purchase of this equipment, which is a business expense, may allow you to be more responsive to your clients and to better use your time.
- E-mail systems will save time for practitioners who regularly work with other

professionals or who are in large offices. With E-mail any member of the staff can leave messages on another's computer so that, as soon as the computer is turned on, the message is delivered. The security of this system, however, is limited because anyone who has system-level access and knowledge of the E-mail system can read your messages. This can be avoided by using passwords to restrict access.

■ A copy machine is another important time saver to add to your communications equipment. From time to time, patients may ask for a copy of their records. With their signed permission (and assuming that there are no state laws to prohibit it), you can copy their records or a summary for them. You will find many other business reasons for needing a copier.

Personnel

Many therapists choose to work without support staff, contracting with office service organizations for special needs such as billing or answering services. Others may have only one person who is responsible for a variety of tasks. In larger offices and practices with multiple offices, there may be a significant number of employed staff. Although this section cannot attempt to present all of the information needed for personnel management, consider these basic business aspects of staffing your office.

■ Several options for obtaining staff are available in most parts of the United States:

- The practice can become the employer of record and hire individuals to work on a regular basis, either part-time or full-time.
- The practice can contract with individuals to provide specific services (independent contractors). In this case, the practice is not the employer. A contract is prepared specifying what services will be provided and the conditions of the working arrangement. (Your attorney should draw up the contract.)
- The practice that participates in an office-sharing arrangement with other professionals may have access to shared staff. The practice usually is not the employer but contributes to an organization that acts on behalf of all of the members in the shared arrangement.
- The practice can contract with an employment agency that provides staff as needed. Again, the practice is not the employer of record.

■ The advantages of being the employer or directly contracting with individuals is that the practice principals are in full control of who is hired, how they are paid, the evaluation of their work, and all job assignments. The disadvantages of being the employer of record are the responsibilities placed on you by federal and state governments. As an employer, a practice is responsible for the following:

- Withholding and submitting federal and state income taxes. At the end of each year, reports must be filed with the government agencies and the employees provided with W-2 Wage and Tax Statements or a Form 1099 for contract employees.
- Withholding, paying, and submitting social security and Medicare taxes. In addition to computing the amount owed by the employee, the employer contributes an equal amount. Payment must be made when the taxes are incurred (usually every pay day) and reports must be filed quarterly.
- Paying unemployment funds (state and federal), workers' compensation (state), and verifying immigration or naturalization status of all workers.
- Maintenance of all payroll records for a period of 3 years or until the statute of limitations on income tax audits expires.

All of these responsibilities are clearly delineated by the federal and state agencies responsible and are provided to practices that apply for an employer identification number. Complying with the various laws, however, is time consuming, and penalties for failure to follow the proper procedures can be stiff.

■ The advantages of not being the employer of record but obtaining services through the other arrangements mentioned earlier are that the practice avoids the legal requirements for taxes, employee insurance, and record keeping. The service or the individual under contract assumes those responsibilities; your practice simply pays their fees. The disadvantages are loss of control over who is hired, how they are rewarded for their work in the practice, and, perhaps, the assignment of work.

Whatever you decide about staffing your practice, be sure to prepare a procedure manual for each job, even if you are going to do that job yourself. Using this Guidebook as a guide and resource, develop step-by-step guidelines for completing each task in the office. Indicate not only who is to do each task but who is to be contacted if problems arise. Include samples of forms that are used. The manual might also list frequently called telephone numbers, miscellaneous office matters (location of keys, how to reorder forms, how to contact other staff in case of an emergency), or anything that would help the incumbent—whether directly employed by you or shared with others—in completing his or her job. If clear instructions about what is to be done and how well it is to be done are not given to all workers, you cannot hold them accountable for the outcome.

Computers and Management Information Systems

In the past decade, the computer industry shifted its attention from large computer systems suitable only for serving large corporations, government agencies, and educational institutions to PCs that can be used in all businesses, institutions, and personal environments. As a result, the computer systems needed by the average small business or practice are affordable, take up little space, and are easy for new users to understand and operate. Larger practices already have recognized the advantages of automating many of the routine functions of their business operations.

Patient volume, with the resulting overflow of paperwork from billing, claim filing, and collections routines, forced an examination of a computer's potential for reducing overhead expenses and lag time in obtaining payment for services. Contracts with large volume purchasers require management information systems that track utilization, monitor payment, and assure that contractual agreements are fulfilled.

Computers are also an essential tool for making smaller practices—including solo practices—more businesslike. PCs usually provide all of the computing capacity required in a small office, and general business software and special software for mental health professionals is readily available and affordable. This section explains why and how a PC can bring greater efficiency and quality improvement to a smaller practice.

General Office Automation

Psychology is generally thought of as a "cottage industry," yet many psychologists are buying computers to keep up with business and technology. Therapists have found that computers have many uses in solo and small group practices. Here are some benefits of automation:

- Improvement in the quality of patient records, billing, and other office procedures.
- Reduction in claims submission errors and delays, resulting in an increase in cash flow.
- Better information on fees, reimbursement arrangements, and collections percentages that allow you to develop better pricing strategies.
- Easy-to-access information on the characteristics of your patient population, referral patterns, average length of treatment, and most common types of cases you treat. This information can be used to develop marketing plans that will help you attract more patients and get the attention of MCOs with whom you would like to contract.
- Decrease in the amount of time required to enter the same data on several different forms (patient's business record, accounting and billing system, clinical record, etc.).
- Ability to establish new office routines (sending notes to potential referrers, retrieving patients' records by diagnosis or treatment mode to study or establish practice guidelines, reminders of follow-up for recently terminated patients, etc.).
- Ability to establish and monitor quality improvement routines and adhere to them.

If you have no knowledge of computers, selecting a system can be daunting. The best way to begin is not with the computer itself but with some consideration of what you will do with it. Make a list of functions or processes that are important to your practice (patient records, accounting, word processing, etc.). Most practices purchase their first computer to perform routine business functions such as billing, collecting, and insurance processing. Automated accounting and bookkeeping programs (including payroll, check writing, and preparation of standard profit and loss statements) cannot only save time but improve the accuracy of your financial management. After these initial applications of computers, you will find many other uses for your computer: scheduling appointments, writing correspondence and routine reports, and preparing marketing materials and staff manuals, among others.

Accounting and Billing: Small Business Software

The proliferation of PCs in small businesses has raised the standards of common business practices. Small business accounting software, a vital segment of the software market, can handle everything from creating a simple invoice to writing checks to paying employees after calculating tax deductions. One great advantage to putting your books onto a PC is obvious when tax time rolls around and all of your data are immediately accessible without thumbing through check registers, canceled checks, and invoices from vendors. Several well-advertised programs are available that can streamline your financial work. These software packages are sufficiently user-friendly so that anyone familiar with a PC and your business needs can computerize the practice books in a few days.

Claims Processing

For those practitioners who decide to file claims for their clients, claims processing software makes the job easy. The claims software uses information previously recorded through scheduling or patient information software programs or is added at the time of service. Diagnoses and service codes, fees, and dates of service are entered from the keyboard and a hard copy is printed—ready for mailing to the insurance company. Most programs have built-in reminders about proper procedures, thus reducing data entry errors or omissions.

Several major insurance companies offer a service, similar to the now-obsolete telex system, that gives you a special terminal in your office that connects to their main computer for filing claims directly. Or you may use a regular PC with a modem to file claims electronically. Electronic claims processing is a rapidly growing practice; some states have proposed legislation to create a national health care information network that would connect insurance companies, providers, and other participants by data network to lower the cost of claims filing. With electronic billing, you are paid for your services more promptly. Medicare and other major payers are encouraging electronic billing.

Quality Improvement: On-Line Computer Networks

As a clinical tool, a PC has equally impressive potential. The growing demand placed on the practicing psychologist by purchasers, insurance companies, and MCOs for objective outcome data is making the use of computers imperative for future success. There are many database programs, from simple to complex, that can help you organize the data you have on client satisfaction, treatment protocols, and practice guidelines. Using a computer to record and analyze these data can vastly expand your knowledge of your practice and enhance its efficacy. The quality improvement suggestions in this chapter can be implemented much more readily by using an automated system.

With a PC and an inexpensive modem, you can access an enormous amount of data on international networks that connect to giant information hubs at universities and government institutions. Professional journals and other periodicals, clinical research data, and other databases of professional interest are also available. Although this Guidebook emphasizes the business side of an automated office, you can use your computer for clinical work as well. A publication of the American Psychological Association, *Computer Use in Psychology*, lists more than 850 software programs in four categories: academic software (classroom or laboratory use), clinical software (useful for some client treatment), statistics and research aids, and psychological testing programs. Some of the programs may be appropriate for your practice.

Basic Hardware Considerations

After you have decided how you want to use your computer, you can select appropriate and compatible software. Another publication from the American Psychological Association, *Hardware, Software, and the Mental Health Professional: The Complete Guide to Office Computerization*, describes hundreds of software programs from which to choose. The book has tables that indicate the comprehensiveness of programs (some will perform all financial management functions; others are limited to a few functions), capacity, and flexibility. And the description of each program describes the hardware requirements, the price of the software, and the installation, training, and ongoing support provided by the software producer.

The basic equipment that you need to set up a single computer is listed below; some systems are sold as packages, including several of the basics, whereas other units are sold separately:

- Keyboard, mouse, and other input devices
- Central processing unit (CPU): This is what most people call the computer — the microprocessor, integrated circuits, memory chips, and expansion boards where the instructions to process data, control and operate the programs, and perform necessary input–output functions are stored and executed.
- Data storage device: The most common storage devices are floppy disks, hard disks, and compact disks. These devices are usually an integral part of the CPU.
- Monitor: A video screen on which the work being performed can be displayed.
- Fax board: A device that permits the computer to send and receive fax messages.
- Modem: Allows transmission of data from one computer to another over telephone lines.
- Printer: The output device. Dot matrix and inkjet printers are generally speedy and provide good draft copy, but in some cases they lack the resolution needed to produce "typewriter-quality" print. Daisy wheel printers are slow but, along with dot matrix printers, are good if you need to print several copies. Inkjets are used often as portable printers. Laser printers print letter-quality copy and do it rapidly.

Cost

The cost of your initial system will vary widely on the basis of the equipment you purchase and the amount of software you need. In estimating the cost of total office automation, obtain an estimate on all of the following costs:

- Hardware: purchase price or lease payments for computer, monitor, keyboard, disks, supplies, printers, and modem.
- Software: purchase price, lease payments, or custom design of applications programs.
- Data conversion: cost of converting your present records to a new system. Most practices do not convert records on terminated patients, so there is little added cost of converting patient records. Converting financial information, however, may require extra wages for data entry clerks or overtime for office staff.
- Site preparation: cost of tables, chairs, additional space, electric outlets, and wiring for terminals, antistatic materials, power surge control units, fire protection, and so on. In most small offices these costs will be minimal, but you need to figure them into the overall costs.
- Maintenance contracts: You may choose to contract for maintenance for both the hardware and software that you purchase (usually estimated at 15% of original cost).

A note of caution: The highest cost in computerizing your office is not included in this list—it is training. The time required to teach you and your staff to operate the equipment, learn the programs, and become proficient will cost you far more than the other elements.

If cost is an issue for you, consider the cost of not establishing good business practices (which includes automation). Remember how much of your billable time you spend looking up phone numbers, checking your schedule, searching for clients' insurance information, retyping a letter just like the one you wrote to another person, and keeping track of who owes you money and for how long. All of this and much more of what you do countless times a day can and should be automated.

Technical Support

Buying a computer is similar to buying a car. There are many options for the initial purchase, but service and repairs are equally important. Most people who know little or nothing about car repairs choose to buy a car from a dealer who can help choose the best model and handle repairs. It is the same in the PC market. Those more adventurous or technically inclined can buy a computer through the mail. The quality of mail order equipment is usually equal to the quality of machines you buy from a dealer. Whether you buy from a dealer or through a mail order house, be sure that you check their reputations. In addition to checking with previous customers, you might want to look through the computer journals for reviews and ratings by experts of the various computer products. And whether you ordered from a catalog or bought everything locally, check the vendor for technical support. Frequently, technical support for 1–3 years is included in the purchase price.

You can buy fixed-price technical support contracts for the services of a technician who will perform repairs on- or off-site, with delivery or without. Be sure that you investigate the service before you buy. You may choose to work with a consultant. There are consultants—students, independent consultants, and employees of large dealerships and consulting firms—who will set up a single computer with software, train you to operate it, and handle repairs. If you do not want to spend your time learning all about computers and fixing them when they fail, this can be an attractive arrangement. Remember, when a PC breaks down, the do-it-yourself approach can be a black hole for consuming your time, and your time is valuable. The best place way to look for technical consulting or support is to check the classified ads in the newspapers and check with colleagues who already have PCs.

Many of the software companies listed in *Hardware, Software, and the Mental Health Professional* indicate that they will install the software that you purchase and train the users. Usually, such services are an additional cost. Most hardware and software companies provide telephone trouble-shooting services at little or no cost. Be sure you ask what services are provided for the purchase price.

Quality Improvement

As competition for health care dollars increases, the quest for quality also increases. Payers of mental health benefits demand that their providers have systems for assuring and maintaining quality of services and that they can prove their superiority. Creating such systems is not an easy task.

Many companies in the United States have initiated total quality management (TQM) or continuous quality improvement programs to involve all employees and managers in accepting responsibility for making continuous improvements in the quality of the company's services and products in order to satisfy customers' needs. A customer is anyone who is the recipient of a product or service, whether he or she is inside or outside the firm. TQM advocates doing the "right" thing the first time and every time thereafter, thus giving a company an edge over competitors.

The principles of TQM also apply to operating a mental health services practice. The customers are your clients, those in your referral base, others in the practice, and the external agencies and payers with which the practice does business. The process of quality improvement (QI) involves collecting data, measuring the data against professional standards or guidelines, and devising activities to bring future measurements closer to the accepted standards. Where standards do not exist, practitioners must begin collecting data to develop practice guidelines or treatment protocols.

Ongoing measurement of the efficacy of various treatments is enabled by an effective management information system. By using information systems that track the care given to clients in the past, a good practice can define the best procedure to follow, measure whether the outcome differs when one treatment regimen is followed rather than another, and determine what additional services, tests, and referrals to other specialists are truly useful. Similar systems are used by many third-party payers for retrospective studies (UR) and prospectively (QA or quality management).

Measuring Client Satisfaction

Other health care organizations can measure customer or client satisfaction, in part by the number of clients who complete a course of treatment and the number who refer friends and relatives to the practice. In mental health care, a more direct approach is needed because, regardless of your skill as a clinician, many of your clients will make only one or a very few visits before self-terminating therapy. Direct questioning is the best approach to determine how clients rate your services. Questionnaires and surveys are the most frequently used method of assessing customer satisfaction.

- In general, written questionnaires or surveys sent through the mail that people can complete at their leisure yield the best results. Mail surveys are inexpensive and generally produce the greatest amount of responses. Other techniques are telephone surveys using a consistent set of questions for each call, personal interviews, or surveys that are designed to be completed while the client is in the office.

  The questions should include information about the practice's response to the client (e.g., How long did it take to get an appointment? Were the staff courteous and helpful?) as well as the client's assessment of his or her progress. You might include some of the questions that employers and payers will be asking: Is the client leading a productive life—back to work, functioning well in daily activities, and so forth? Did the outpatient therapy or substance abuse treatment prevent hospitalization? Does the client feel better about himself or herself? Did he or she reach reasonable goals that let him or her resume normal activities? In other words, from the client's perspective, did the therapy work?

  Whenever possible, design a format using multiple-choice questions instead of open-ended questions. People tend to check off items on a list more readily than they make written comments. Also, the forced choice of selected items makes compilation of the responses much easier. A few open-ended questions at the end of a structured survey may yield useful comments.

- Keep the survey short and simple. Make it easy for people to respond by supplying a self-addressed, stamped return envelope or ask them to deposit their responses in a marked box in the reception area.

- If your customers include other practitioners, EAP staff, or physicians, design a short questionnaire for them to complete to help you see how you are rated by your referrers. Follow the same guidelines as for patient satisfaction surveys.

- If you have a contract with an MCO, inquire about their satisfaction survey procedures. Many of them survey their members annually, and the questionnaires sometimes assess individual service providers like you.

When you have collected information from your customers, analyze the data to see whether there is any consistency in the comments. Do not be surprised if you receive a few negative comments. And do not change your practices on the basis of a few negative statements. Look at the majority of responses. If some aspects of your practice are clearly more desirable than others, accent the positive and correct or amend those that most clients do not like.

Practice Guidelines and Clinical Protocols

Mental health care does not have rigid standards by which to judge the efficacy of treatment or successful patient outcomes. Although research on patient outcomes continues, other avenues are more helpful in improving the quality of mental health care.

Using common business techniques to gather information about how patients are evaluated, treated, and cared for after treatment helps to improve the care for future patients. You can improve the clinical side of your practice by recording what you do with each patient and comparing the results when patients with the same diagnosis or type of problem are treated differently. The data you gather in a business context and for business purposes will not be in the same depth that you are likely to be used to when gathering data for clinical purposes. Yet, this abbreviated and focused form of data gathering is critical for competing in today's marketplace.

Here are some hints for establishing your own QI system:

- Create a procedure for systematically recording information about patients in the clinical record. Try to follow the same procedure and format for each patient. Whenever possible, specify treatment goals, use standardized measurement instruments and tests, and use agreed-on measures of functionality.

  - Standardize the intake interview. Create forms to capture the patient's history and presenting problems in a consistent manner. Specify the patient's expectations for treatment.
  - Note the results of all standardized tests.
  - Use a standard format for summarizing each session for the patient's record. If possible, ask the patient to describe his or her progress and record the responses.
  - At the end of treatment, review the original goals with your patient and obtain his or her progress rating.
  - Develop a follow-up schedule for each diagnosis, type of problem, or other method of categorizing your patients. Send a questionnaire to each patient at the scheduled time or call each one for an informal update on his or her progress.

- Analyze the data gathered in the process listed previously. First, categorize your patients in a manner that is meaningful to you (e.g., by diagnosis, by presenting situation, by length of treatment, etc.). Track the cases with the greatest degree of success in reaching the specified goals. Note the commonalities and differences in the way you treated those patients: number of treatments, pattern of visits, timing of interventions, treatment sites and settings, modalities, and so forth. When a clear pattern exists, describe the pattern carefully and follow it for all similar patients. Continue to review the patterns and change your procedures accordingly as better ones emerge. Because QI requires that every case be scrutinized, review every case in this manner.

■ From the QI data, develop the following statistics:

- The average number of visits for each of the categories of patients that you are tracking (total number of visits by category divided by the number of patients in that category).
- Average cost per case by category (average number of visits by category multiplied by your per visit rate if that rate is constant; if not, calculate the cost of all of the care given in the category divided by the number of cases).
- Success ratio by category (number of patients who successfully met therapy goals divided by number of patients in that category). *Success* might be defined as reaching 75% of the goals stated at the initial visit or by the patient's perception or statement of his or her progress at the terminal visit.
- Average length of stay by diagnosis for patients who are hospitalized.

Use these statistics when competing for managed care contracts, compare them with data that you receive from third parties to ensure that their statistics present the same picture of your practice as the facts that you have gathered, and discuss your outcomes with the principals in your practice or peer review groups in which you are active. As mental health services professionals continue their research on standards of treatment and outcomes measures, compare their findings with the practice guidelines that you constructed from your QI program.

Managed Care Processes

MCOs, with their interest in controlling cost and access to health care, gather data on the providers in their systems to determine which providers meet their standards. Historically, they have measured and monitored the amount of services delivered and cost of providing care. These measures often determine whether a provider is solicited to serve on the panel of providers or, after becoming a member of a panel, whether he or she is asked to continue to serve on the panel. This process is often referred to as "economic credentialing" because a major factor in the review is the comparison of the treatment costs of one practitioner with another. Most of the data collected and used in these reviews are derived from hospital records and claims that have been filed. Efforts at credentialing providers on the basis of their cost effectiveness typically fail to take into account the quality of care delivered or the nature of the population being treated. Some innovative MCOs, however, are beginning to place greater emphasis on provider quality rather than cost.

UR is often viewed by practitioners as an intrusion on their care of the patient, particularly if the person conducting the review is not a trained mental health care professional. The APA has drafted model legislation designed to address many of the problems with the way UR has traditionally been applied to psychologists. Professionals may not accept that practitioner profiles—comparison of their cost and treatment modalities—used to compare therapists are appropriate measures of quality. It is, however, a common third-party practice that is not likely to be discontinued. You should look for ways to include some of the resulting information in your QI program.

The UR process usually includes precertification for your services prior to treatment, review of your treatment plan, administrative review to determine whether your practice is adhering to the regulations, discharge planning, and occasionally an audit of your books and records.

The following are some suggestions for working UR into your QI plan:

- Precertification usually occurs after your first visit with the client. Your telephone contact with the reviewer should establish the need for this patient to receive treatment and to establish your credentials for providing that treatment. You can learn what benefits the reviewer's organization covers in its insurance program, how they regard your credentials and history, and how to best articulate your precertification requests in the future. Some experts suggest that you record some of your conversations with reviewers (and tell them that you are doing so) so that you have documentation of the decisions reached and approval to proceed. One approach might be to ask permission to tape the conversation so that you can have a record of what the managed care company needs. Your aim is to provide—within legal limits—the data needed to approve treatment for your patient. You also have a record to study to determine how you might improve your ability to conduct the precertification interview. Keep records on what you learn about this part of the process so that you can improve your next interaction with the reviewer.

- After you have approval to begin treatment of the client, develop an initial treatment plan. Most organizations are interested in acute problem resolution and, if necessary, coordination of long-term care. They prefer short-term, symptom-oriented care. Clearly, if that is not the best way to treat a patient, you have an ethical responsibility to try to convince the reviewer that another approach is likely to yield better results. Demonstrate to the reviewer that you understand his or her responsibility to ensure that treatment is focused on treating the immediate problem.

- Apply for extensions of your treatment plan when necessary. Explain why the patient needs additional treatment in jargon-free language. After some experience, you can include in your QI process a list of reasons for extensions that have proved acceptable.

- When the patient appears ready to terminate his or her care, you may be asked to help with discharge planning by designing or justifying aftercare. You should specify what type of follow-up is needed and the schedule. Your QI plan should include suggested follow-up routines for each type of patient you see (manic–depressive, chronic pain, personality disorders, phobias, etc.).

- Each third-party payer supplies a provider manual containing all of its administrative regulations at the time you sign a contract. Administrative reviews are generally conducted by business office staff who are interested not in the treatment of the patient but in how billing and other practices have been carried out. Your business office staff should be able to handle this review on your behalf. However, if you become involved, review the manual before talking with the reviewer so that you can use their terminology. Read the administrative regulations carefully when you first get your contracts. Often, you can establish standard office procedures that will cover most third-party requirements. The few regulations that are unique to a certain plan will be easier to identify and accommodate if you already have a routine that covers most of the rules.

■ Involvement with third parties can result in an audit of your accounts and patient records. Review your own books and patient records on a regular basis, or ask a colleague to review them for you in exchange for your audit of his or her practice. Be sure you have your patient's consent for the audit or limit your audit to the verification that appropriate forms are completed and in the file. (See the Financial Management for self-audit and Practice Guidelines and Clinical Protocols sections earlier in this chapter.)

Case management is another method of monitoring the care provided to a patient and the attendant cost. Usually, case management is concurrent with care and more often conducted by mental health professionals. The case manager reviews not only the treatment plans and progress of the patient but also the setting in which treatment is given. Frequently, the case manager can approve home care, aftercare, halfway houses, and other community-based settings on your recommendation.

Marketing

Although marketing is not usually considered a business system, it is a critical element in operating a successful practice. Practices do not grow by chance; they increase because they offer services that suit the needs and interests of a segment of the population.

Many professionals equate marketing with public relations or selling. Although some elements of both may be present in marketing, they are more often activities performed to reach a specific marketing goal. A formal definition of marketing is the analysis, planning, implementation, and control of carefully formulated programs designed to bring about voluntary exchanges of values for purposes of achieving organizational objectives. In psychological practices, the values exchanged are your professional services for an appropriate fee. Marketing relies heavily on designing the products and services of a practice in terms of the target market's needs and desires and on using effective pricing, communication, and distribution to inform, motivate, and service the markets. Marketing is what psychologists do best— building relationships and influencing change.

This section presents a brief look at marketing your practice on the basis of the goals of the practice and the needs of various clients. The suggestions for marketing activities should be selected after careful consideration of all of the elements in the marketing process.

The Marketing Process

The marketing process is remarkably compatible with strategic planning; when you determine your goals for the practice, you can easily identify the targets for your marketing. For example, if you need to increase the number of private-pay patients in your practice in order to have a balanced patient mix, you will need to perform some marketing activities that will introduce you to likely new contacts. You might develop a campaign to meet with ministers, home health nurses, and Meals-on-Wheels personnel to identify ways in which you could serve their clients or the families of their clients. If you are comfortable with public speaking, your activities might include presenting workshops or giving presentations on mental health topics to community groups. Or you might agree to write a column for a local newspaper or the newsletters of companies in your neighborhood. All of these activities would fit with the goal to increase the number of private patients.

The targets for marketing your services often fall into three general categories: contacts with prospective patient sources, additional referrals (either new sources or more referrals from present sources), and large-volume purchasers (insurance companies, MCOs, employers, EAPs). Different activities will be needed for each of these target audiences because each places a different value on your services on the basis of its needs.

To market your services effectively, you must find out what customers need and want and then demonstrate to the customer how you can fulfill that need. It is incumbent on the "seller" to motivate the buyer to buy; selling works best when it is based on specific needs of the buyer.

Much of the work that needs to be done to demonstrate how your practice can match your customer's need was completed in the strategic planning chapter using the PATs (see the Appendix). The analysis of your practice, the environment, local market, and current client base is the foundation for all of your marketing activities. Keep in mind your responses to the data gathering forms in the PATs as you look at the steps in developing your market activities.

1. Review the market for your services. You might choose to skim the first two chapters of the Guidebook and note local adaptations of the trends. Review the Area Market Data, Referral Base, and Patient–Payer Profiles sections in the PATs.

2. Analyze your practice to determine what you have to offer. Consider your training and education, specialties, credentials, and reputation. The Practice Record, the Fact Sheet, and Quality Improvement sections of the PATs will provide the information you need. But do not forget the business aspects of your services. Review the cost per case, average number of visits by diagnosis, and efficiency measures that may set your practice apart from the competition.

3. Set goals for your marketing plan for 1 year on the basis of the needs of your practice. Perhaps you will select one target in each of the categories listed previously: new contacts, referral base, and volume purchasers. For example, your goals might be to

• Maintain the present level of private-pay patients in my practice (i.e., find a replacement for every terminating private-pay patient).

- Increase my referral base of primary care physicians by contacting and working with five physicians in the next year.
- Obtain a contract with one new volume purchaser in the next 6 months.

4. Research the needs for mental health services of your target audiences. For a large employer, for example, find out as much about the company as you can—products and services, demographics of the employee and dependent population, organizational culture, related human resources programs and activities, and so forth. This research helps you to match your products to the client's needs.

5. Develop support materials for the marketing efforts. Some of the support materials must be in print to be distributed to potential clients. Others may be for your personal use such as workshop or presentation outlines.

6. Select marketing activities that will help you reach your practice goals and make a list of what you need to do and when. For example, if your first project needs to be the preparation of print material for your sales efforts to an MCO, your activities might include the following list:

- Spend 3 hours in Week 1 researching and completing a practice capabilities statement.
- Devote 2 hours in Weeks 2 and 3 discussing the capabilities statement and your marketing approach with a trusted colleague or friend.
- Commit 6 hours during the first 4 weeks researching MCOs in your community and selecting one that you would like to attempt to join as a panel member. Mark your "things to do" list with the marketing activities that you plan to accomplish and indicate the deadline for each. Marketing is most successful when it becomes a daily or weekly exercise, a part of your good business routines.

7. Every quarter (at the same time that you conduct an overall review of your practice and its finances), review your marketing activities and goals. Make adjustments as needed if your first strategies did not work out as well as you expected. But do not quit. Marketing is an ongoing process.

Measures of Effectiveness and Efficiency

Part of your marketing effort—regardless of the "purchaser"—will include statements about the therapeutic effectiveness of your practice in working with clients. In some cases, such as marketing to MCOs, EAPs, or larger groups that you would like to join, you will also need to show evidence of business efficiency. Here are some ideas that can help you develop a record of your competence and incorporate it into your marketing plan.

Outcomes measures and comparisons

■ Track your cases by diagnosis or type of counseling. Aggregate the cases in a way that supports your presentation to your client. For example, assume that you dealt with 20 cases of substance abuse: 5 patients with bipolar disorders, 12 families in distress, and 4 spousal abuse cases during the past year. In presenting your credentials to an EAP that is primarily concerned with substance abuse, you would stress that substance abuse cases represent the largest number of your clients. If, however, you were marketing to a group practice that is seeking a therapist with broad-based therapy skills, you might emphasize the variety of cases that you have handled. And if you were seeking a practice that primarily helps dysfunctional families, you would demonstrate that a majority of your cases (substance abuse, family counseling, and spousal abuse) deal with aspects of family dysfunction. (Use the forms in the Quality Improvement section of the PATs to begin your tracking.)

- Determine the average number of visits for each major diagnostic group you have served. In managed care and EAPs, this figure is crucial because they place a premium on short-term problem resolution. For other clients or prospective partners, this figure allows a comparison with other therapists dealing with similar diagnoses or problems.

- If your patients are hospitalized, determine the average length of stay in the hospital for each diagnosis. Most hospitals can provide you with this figure along with data that compare the stays of your patients with those of other therapists' patients with the same diagnosis. MCOs and multispecialty groups will compare your profile with their standards and other providers.

- For each diagnosis, compute the average cost per case. Wherever possible, try to obtain data on the overall cost of each case, not just your charges. For example, if you routinely refer types of cases for testing and evaluation services, find out how much that costs on average and show it as part of your presentation to prospective clients.

- Define therapeutic success for each diagnosis or type of case you treat and specify how success will be measured. This is a very difficult task but important in demonstrating your abilities, comparing the services of one therapy group with another, or developing practice parameters for use by all principals in a group. Can you determine and measure success by valid tests? Is the ability to return to work, school, or other activities success? Is the client's personal statement that he or she has attained the personal goals set for therapy an acceptable measure? In presenting your practice to a potential buyer, explain your success measure and indicate how effective you have been in meeting that standard.

- Document your normal procedures and processes for treating patients. State how you conduct the initial patient evaluation. List the tests and measurements that you usually use with each diagnostic category. Indicate how you determine whether the client should remain under your care and when you would refer for specialty care. What criteria do you use to decide whether a patient needs individual care or can be properly incorporated into a group? Customers— particularly volume buyers—look for signs that your practice follows each patient in an organized, businesslike fashion.

Techniques for determining business efficiency

- If you are processing insurance claims for your patients, they should be filed within 3 days of the visit. If claims are not being filed within the 3-day period, change the procedures so that claims are a priority or get more help. In some cases, when you are seeing a patient frequently, you may choose to send claim forms at the end of each month. Clients should be made aware of how soon after their visit you will file their claim.

- Review randomly selected insurance claims forms to ensure that coding is being entered properly. Using information from the patient record, check the diagnostic codes, the procedure codes, and the amounts billed for each procedure. Schedule a monthly or quarterly coding audit. Your accuracy in filing claims is as important to your client as it is to your financial operations. No client wants to be involved in a hassle over insurance claims.

- Insurance claims that have not been paid within 30 days of their submission should be followed-up. Check to see whether your claims are being aggressively pursued. If you are filing claims yourself, set aside time at the end of every month for resubmitting claims or requesting a review of those that are underpaid. Unpaid claims should be treated as other overdue bills. Let your clients know that you investigate unpaid claims made on their behalf.

- Calculate your overhead rate (see the Business Management section of the PATs for the method of calculation). Although this is not a figure that clients need to know, you may wish to indicate that you are able to keep your overhead expenses low because of your regular review of expenses. Low overhead for you can mean lower prices for your clients.

Marketing support materials. Most therapists find it helpful to develop support materials for their marketing programs using the information that you have about your practice: products, services, credentials, history, prices, and quality measures. No single document will be appropriate for all sales contacts but, having prepared some basic documents, you can quickly adapt the materials to suit the needs of potential clients.

Your practice will regularly contact clients, potential purchasers, and other businesses. Be sure that all print materials represent you well. Have a graphic designer prepare a design for letterheads and envelopes, bills and statements, forms, reports, proposals, and any other print formats that you plan to use. Or choose a design available from a printer, stationery company, or software program. Make sure that the design and the colors project the image of your practice. Make up business cards not only for the principals in the practice but for key support staff who may be dealing with others on your behalf.

The Client Information Brochure, discussed further in the Supplementary Materials following this chapter, can be used in some sales presentations. The brochure should contain a description of your practice and a list of procedures that make your practice efficient and effective for your patients. If you prepare the brochure from the client's perspective, it can be used as a handout (along with your business card) whenever you make contact with a new group or potential referral source.

Many companies, consulting organizations, and practices develop a document called a *capabilities statement*. This statement is a carefully drafted, concise description of your practice, products, services, and abilities. It should contain at least the following items:

- A restatement of the primary goal, product, service, or specialty of the practice that would be meaningful to a client. For example, "The Elm Street Clinic, serving the greater metropolitan area, was established more than 10 years ago to provide help through counseling to victims of violence, abuse, and dysfunctional families" or "City Psychological Center was founded in 1984 as a partnership of L. Martin Williams, MD, and Sarah Walston, MD, to facilitate the founders' interests in career counseling, aptitude testing, and the study of mid-career changes."

- Brief descriptions of the products and services and how they are delivered. In a multispecialty practice, tell the client the types of cases handled and styles of counseling used. In a specialty practice, describe the appropriate details. In the example of the career counseling clinic just noted, you might explain the testing procedures, the role of the person being counseled, the length of time required, and follow-up procedures after counseling.

- Staff qualifications and experience. An overall statement in the body of the capabilities statement outlining the types of experience that might interest the customer should be appended with brief résumés of key staff.

- Facilities and office or clinic location. Depending on the nature of your practice, you might want to emphasize the ambiance of the practice, its convenient location, or both.

- Unique or innovative services or measures of quality. Briefly describe any unusual elements of your practice.

The capabilities for many practices will not exceed two or three pages plus appended résumés. For larger practices and clinics, the statement might be five or six pages. These statements are often printed as brochures or inserts in presentation folders. Although they need not be fancy or expensive, your capabilities statement must be well written, concise, and attractively presented. If you are making a formal proposal to a client, a folder with the capabilities statement followed by the proposal makes a good package.

If you plan to make numerous proposals to other organizations or buyers, consider developing a standard proposal format. Once such a format—along with some of the "boilerplate" text that is often required in proposals—is filed in your word-processor, it will be easy to quickly prepare proposals for new clients.

Many therapists have public speaking and workshop presentation skills that can enhance marketing activities. Both are particularly useful in making contact with public groups that might be sources of private-pay patients. In order to obtain appropriate engagements, prepare a two-page description of your speech or workshop; discuss the content, benefits, general schedule or timing, and make sure that your name, address and phone number are prominently displayed. Distribute the description whenever you make new contacts or send it by direct mail to groups that you have identified as potential sources of patients. Develop audiovisuals and handouts to accompany your presentation.

To prepare these documents—client brochure, capabilities statement, proposal format (if needed), and workshop and presentation descriptions—you will need to put yourself in the client role to determine what should be included. (See the Outline for a Proposal to a Managed Care Organization at the end of this chapter for an example of how the basic documents might be incorporated into a formal proposal.)

Marketing activities. The following are some suggestions for marketing activities that may be appropriate for your practice. Some clearly are designed to enhance your referral base; others are ways to build a private patient base. Be sure that you have outlined your marketing goals before you select any of these activities. Choosing activities because they look like fun or are particularly easy to perform may not help.

- Make a list of all the people and organizations that can be expected to continue to refer to you. Compose two print pieces that can be mailed to each individual or company on the list:

  - A simple "thank you" for past referrals and a request for future consideration.
  - A brief practice announcement—a description of your services, your location, hours, and phone number, specialty or preferred treatment modality, and any other information that would make it easy for the referrer to remember you and to contact you when he or she wishes to make a referral. This statement should be suitable for giving to a prospective client. Send more than one copy to those offices that are frequent referrers so that they can give a copy to the client whom they are referring.

- Looking at the list of individuals and practices that refer to you, consider whether there are health care professionals or organizations that you logically could expect to refer clients to you but who have not sent clients in the past. Make a "new contacts" list of the names and addresses of potential referral sources. For example, if there are several primary care physicians in the area who may have patients suffering from depression, you could expect referrals from them. If they are not sending clients to you, add them to your new contacts list. Compose a simple introductory letter explaining your services and your availability. Mail a copy, along with the practice statement, to each of the people on the list. Remember that the referral list should include not only other mental health professionals and local physicians but other health workers as well. Often, the first health care worker to hear about a person's mental health problem is not in a mental health care field.

- When you receive a referral—particularly one from a new source—keep the referrer informed with a progress report on the patient without breaching confidentiality. A note or phone call that indicates you and the patient have made contact and are entering a relationship is probably sufficient information. Keep in mind that a satisfied client is your best advertising with other professionals.

- Welcome new health care professionals who set up practice in your area. Let them know about your business, offer to help them in setting up their offices by recommending vendors and services in the community, answering questions about the neighborhood, and so on. Visit those who might be good referral sources. Be sure to take your business cards and practice statements.

- Express your appreciation for every referral you receive. Cards, notes, letters, and phone calls cost little but make a big impression. Include in the office procedures for your receptionist (or yourself) a reminder to send your thanks after each new referral. Your thanks can be expressed in the same communication as the progress report you send.

- Personal contact is far more effective—and more time consuming—than contacts through the mail. Find ways to approach potential referrers as you go about your other professional activities. Always carry business cards and, if possible, have a supply of the practice statements with you whenever you leave your office. Check your referral log before each professional meeting you attend so that you can remember to personally thank those who have sent clients to you. Whenever you meet a potential new referral source, get his or her business card and follow up immediately with a personal letter. Describe your practice interests, state clearly that you appreciate referrals, and include some practice statements.

- Enhancing the prominence of your practice by presenting a paper at a scientific meeting, taking in a new partner, giving a speech to a community group, or participating in any number of other events is likely to gain referrals. To capitalize on those activities, send a letter outlining the new skills that you acquired through continuing education or a copy of an article or paper you have written to all of the members of your network. Let your network know of your accomplishments, not to boast but to inform.

- Be a good referrer when it is your turn to send a client to another practitioner. Choose providers whom you respect. Provide them with appropriate information about your referral. Thank them for any advice and assistance they give to the client.

- Your referral list probably contains the names of several EAPs and their staff members. They may be good referral sources even if you are not on their panel of providers. Remember that companies that do not have formal EAPs still may have employees who need your help. Contact the health, personnel, or human resources offices of the companies in your area to let them know of your services. Ask to be placed on their lists for referrals. Even if they do not have a formal referral program, they may have an informal system of suggesting therapists for employees with problems. Offer to provide a free service, such as a lecture or discussion of the tensions of raising children, how to manage personal stress, the emotional problems of dealing with aging parents, to introduce yourself to employees. The contact with the company and its employees may lead to many new clients.

- Be active in your community and encourage your staff to be active too. In professional groups, volunteer work, hobbies and sports, and social engagements let people know what you do and how you can be contacted.

- Become involved in local schools. Some psychologists specialize in treating children and adolescents; others may be more interested in treating the parents and teachers of school-age children.

- Participate in local health events such as health screenings and health fairs. Volunteer to help the organizers or set up a booth to distribute information about mental health issues.

- Make sure that your practice is listed prominently in the Yellow Pages of the local telephone directory. Even regular referral sources may have misplaced your phone number or may not know your exact location. A small advertisement that provides space for you to describe your specialty, show your logo, and list your qualifications may attract clients to your practice. Be sure that the text of your ad does not promise what you cannot supply but if, for example, you can provide same-day appointments, say so. State facts only, not opinions, and do not give guarantees.

- If there are Welcome Wagons, Newcomers Clubs, or a local Chamber of Commerce in your community, provide your practice statement to them for distribution. New residents who are under stress from their move or adjustment may want your help.

- Advertise your practice through public speaking and writing. If you are good at public speaking, contact local civic organizations and offer to speak on mental health issues. Local TV and radio shows often like to have an expert available to comment on psychological issues in the news. Volunteer by writing to the local stations and giving them your credentials. Write an occasional column for the local newspaper. Volunteer to write a column for the newsletters that a local employer distributes to its employees and their dependents. Keep the language simple and choose topics that are of general interest or are timely. And, of course, be sure your name appears in the byline.

Professional Consultants

Nearly all practitioners—whether new to practice or experienced—need some professional services. As noted, you may wish to contract with management consultants to help you establish your initial practice or to assist you with specific problems that arise during its operation. Perhaps a marketing expert could help your group in examining options for new services that would help the practice grow. An accountant can assist you in framing your financial policies and perhaps perform your bookkeeping and file your tax returns. An attorney may be necessary to help you with creating the legal entity for your practice—sole proprietor, partnership, or corporation—or drawing up employment contracts. The growing importance of computers in all types of businesses suggests that a computer or management information systems specialist might be another valuable source of business help. Finding the right consultant requires some investigation. (See Choosing and Using Consultants at the end of this chapter.)

You will probably need consultants for short-term assistance to solve specific problems. An accountant and a lawyer should, however, be selected partly because they are willing to work with you over time. The accountant's role might include helping to establish your bookkeeping routines, reviewing your books on a quarterly basis and conducting an audit at year's end, filing your tax returns, and financial planning.

When you are starting out, consult an attorney about the proper legal entity for the type of practice you wish to establish (see chapter 4). In addition to drawing up the papers for your practice (partnership agreement, articles of incorporation, office-sharing arrangement), you may need help in obtaining the licenses, provider numbers, leases, and employment contracts needed for your practice. Ask your attorney about insurance coverage—both professional liability and business coverage—to protect you from losses (see the section on business insurance considerations earlier in this chapter.) Meet regularly with your attorney—perhaps two to four times each year—to update him or her on the operation of your practice as well as to obtain answers to specific legal questions you have. An ongoing relationship with and an understanding of your business and professional goals will help your attorney provide routine guidance as well as advice during crises that you may face with clients.

Summary

The changing marketplace, competition with other providers, and the need to protect individual practices from these uncertainties suggest a need for practices to adopt and maintain standard, proven business practices. Maintaining the personalized, caring service image of traditional psychological practices while adding processes to attain efficiency and effectiveness is a daunting task. This chapter has provided a framework for beginning that task.

Chapter 6
Supplementary
Materials

Tips for the Practitioner:

- Social security number and driver's license number can be useful if you need to trace an individual who is delinquent in paying his or her bills.
- Do not accept a post office box number as the only way to contact someone. Ask for the address and phone number of a friend or relative who can get in touch with your patient if needed.
- If your client is a minor in your state, be sure to obtain information about the party responsible for paying for treatment.
- For marketing purposes, you might want to add a question about how your patient was referred to you (or how they heard about you).

Sample Patient Information Sheet

Patient: _____

Last name   First name   Middle

_____

Social security number (optional)   Driver's license number (optional)

_____

Home Address   Street   Apt. #   City   State   Zip code

_____

Home phone number   Work phone number

_____

Name of employer   Occupation

_____

Address   Street   Suite   City   State   Zip code

Spouse: _____

Name   Work phone number   Birthdate

Spouse's Employer _____

Payment method: _____

Cash   Check   Credit card

Insurance: _____

Insurance company   Subscriber no.   Policy no.

_____

Insurance company   Subscriber no.   Policy no.

_____

Workers Compensation   Carrier Medicaid no.   Medicare no.

Responsible party: Complete the section below if you are not the patient but are responsible for the bill.

_____

Responsible party

_____

Relationship to patient

_____

Address   Street   Suite #   City   State   Zip code

_____

Home phone   Work phone number

_____

Employer

Signature _____

(Patient, parent, legal guardian, or responsible party)

Authorization for Release of Information and Records

TO: _____
    (Practitioner, hospital, etc.)

I have been informed that under _____ (state) law, communications between a patient and his or her psychologist are privileged and may not be disclosed by the psychologist unless the patient consents. I also have been informed that patient records maintained by a psychologist may not be disclosed to third parties except with the patient's consent or through legal process.

Please check one of the following:

_____ I hereby authorize you to provide copies of all my patient records to _____ (primary care physician, other health care professional, insurance company). I further authorize you to discuss my case, including my history, treatment, and condition, with _____ (primary care physician, other health care professional, insurance company).

_____ This authorization is only for the limited purpose of releasing information to and discussing my case with _____ (specify). It shall not be deemed a waiver of any privileged communications or confidential information to anyone other than _____ (specify).

This authorization shall remain in effect until revoked by me in writing.

This _____ day of _____, 19____.

_____
Signature

_____   ____ / ____ / ____
Witnessed by   Date

Authorization for Release of Information and Records

TO: Dr. _____
       (Practitioner)

I have been informed that under _____ (state) law, communications between a patient and his or her psychologist are privileged and may not be disclosed by the psychologist unless the patient consents. I also have been informed that patient records maintained by a psychologist may not be disclosed to third parties except with the patient's consent or through legal process.

I hereby authorize Dr. _____ to disclose, release, and/or obtain records to/from

_____ My primary care physician, Dr. _____

_____ My family members as listed _____

_____ My lawyer _____

_____ The person who referred me _____

_____ My previous therapist _____

_____ My insurance company _____

_____ Other _____

This authorization is only for the limited purpose of releasing information to and discussing my case with these individuals or companies for purposes of evaluation and treatment. It shall not be deemed a waiver of any privileged communications or confidential information.

This authorization shall remain in effect until revoked by me in writing.

This _____ day of _____, 19____.

_____
Signature

_____   ____ / ____ / ____
Witnessed by   Date

Authorization for Assignment of Benefits

Medicare

Medicare allows providers to obtain a one-time patient authorization for assignment of benefits if the following requirements are met:

- On the insurance claim form, write, type or stamp "patient's request for payment on file" in the patient signature block (Box 13 on HCFA 1500 claim form).
- Your billing statements sent to patients should clearly indicate (preferably by rubber stamp in red), "Do not use this bill for claiming Medicare benefits. A claim has been or will be submitted to Medicare on your behalf."
- Patient may revoke the authorization and the provider agrees to abide by the patient's wishes. Revoking assignment does not relieve the provider of the responsibility for filing a Medicare patient's claim.
- The patient's signed authorization statement must be available on request for Medicare's investigators. Be sure that the original is firmly attached to the patient's record.

A sample Medicare authorization might read as follows:

I authorize any holder of health or other information about me to be released to the Social Security Administration and Health Care Financing Administration or its intermediaries or carrier any information needed for this or a related Medicare/Medicaid/CHAMPUS claim. I permit a copy of this authorization to be used in place of the original and request payment of insurance benefits either to myself or to the party who accepts assignment. Regulations pertaining to Medicare assignment of benefits apply.

Signature _____   Date _____

Assignment for Other Insurance Carriers

A similar authorization form could be developed for other insurers. Most insurers accept the one-time patient authorization. Be sure to keep the form with the patient's record to substantiate your permission to take assignment of his or her benefits.

Payment Agreement and Assignment of Benefits

My professional fees are based on $ ____ for a standard ____ -minute session. Psychological assessments, consultations, and reports are billed at $ __ per hour. Brief professional services are billed at $ ____ per 15 minutes, or any part thereof, including telephone conversations. Fees may be periodically adjusted and you will be notified in advance of the adjustment.

Payment of accounts are due on receipt of statement of account. Clients are responsible for payment of the total charges shown on the statement of account. We would be pleased to file a claim for your insurance benefits; however, we cannot guarantee payment by the insurance company. If you offer health insurance as complete or partial payment of your fees, we ask that you assign the insurance payments to _____.

Nonpayment of fees will result in termination of professional services and collection activity for amounts owed.

I hereby assign all mental health benefits, including major benefits to which I am entitled, as well as Medicare and other government-sponsored programs, private insurance, and any other health plan to _____, PhD. This assignment will remain in effect until revoked by me in writing. A photocopy of this assignment is to be considered as valid as the original. I understand I am financially responsible for all charges whether paid by said insurance. I hereby authorize Dr. _____ to release all information necessary to secure payment.

_____   _____   __/__/__
Client   Guarantor (if different)   Date

_____   __/__/__
Witness   Date

Sample Medicare Consultation Release Form:
Notice to Medicare Patients

Dear _____ :
  (Patient's name)

It may be beneficial for me to confer with your primary care physician with regard to your psychological treatment or to discuss any medical problems for which you are receiving treatment. In addition, Medicare requires that I notify your physician by telephone or in writing, concerning services that are being provided by me unless you request that notification not be made.

_____
Signature of therapist

Please check one of the following:

__ _____ (practitioner's name) is to contact my primary care physician whose name and address are shown below to discuss treatment that I am receiving while under his or her care and to obtain information concerning my medical diagnosis and treatment.

__ I do not authorize you to contact my primary care physician with regard to the treatment that I am receiving while under your care or to obtain information concerning my medical diagnosis and treatment. I am providing you with the name and address of my primary care physician only for your records.

Please complete all information below:

Primary care physician: _____

Address: _____

_____

Phone: _____

Please print patient's name and address:
_____
_____
_____

Patient's signature _____   Date __/__/__

Payment Agreement

Professional fees are based on $ _____ for a standard _____ -minute session. Psychological assessments, consultations and reports are billed at $ _____ per hour. Brief professional services are billed at $ _____ per 15 minutes, or any part thereof, including telephone conversations. Fees may be periodically adjusted and clients will be notified in advance of the adjustment.

Professional fees will be assessed at the rate of $ _____ per hour, or any part thereof, for any services related to litigation, defense, or other court- or case-related activities. Such activities include interviews, evaluations, research, reports, correspondence, testimony, communication with attorneys, travel, and on-site time. In case of overnight travel, the maximum daily rate will be ___. Incidental expenses for professional services, such as, but not limited to, cost of travel, lodging, and meals, will be billed to the client or his or her attorney.

Payment in full is expected at the time or in advance of services rendered. Statements will be provided for filing insurance claims. Nonpayment of fees will result in termination of professional services and collection activity for amounts owed.

Since professional services are available only through prior scheduling, sessions canceled less than 24 hours in advance are charged at the full rate of the scheduled service.

Any variation from this payment agreement will require a separate written agreement.

I have read this agreement and agree to its terms.

_____   _____   ___/___/___

Client   *Guarantor (if different)*   *Date*

_____   ___/___/___

Witness   *Date*

Insurance Verification

Patient's name _____

Social security number _____

Employer (company name) _____

Name of primary insurance company _____

Telephone number to verify coverage _____

Policyholder's name _____

Group number _____

Identification number _____

Family coverage _____ Individual coverage _____

Does the policy reimburse licensed psychologists? Yes _____   No _____

Outpatient coverage (list all mental health benefits) _____

_____

_____

Percentage covered _____ Maximum reimbursement per visit _____

Deductible $ _____ Has deductible been met for the year? Yes ___   No ___

Contract year (dates) _____

Limits of coverage _____

Date verified _____Insurance contact person _____

Other insurance _____

Client Information Brochure

Distributing a well-written client information brochure is an excellent way to let newcomers to your practice know how your practice operates. The brochure should contain answers to the most frequently asked questions about appointments, emergencies, billing procedures, and other administrative policies. Providing the answers in written form reduces the number of routine phone calls that must be answered by you or your staff. The brochure is a good way to educate long-term patients about your expectations for your relationship with them. Some space in the brochure should be devoted to a description of your practice and the image you wish to present to referrers, potential clients, and current patients.

The following are some of the items you might include in a client information brochure.

- **Type of Practice**
  Be sure to explain clearly the nature of your practice, your training, and experience. Indicate whether your practice is limited to specific types of cases (substance abuse, depression, marital problems), groups of patients (adolescents, women, families, etc.), or therapeutic approaches (Jungian, 12 Step, etc.). If you are a member of a group or partnership and share the patient load from time to time, explain how this benefits the patient. Tell your patients how coverage is provided by others should you be unavailable.
- **Location**
  Be sure to add a map and directions about how to reach your office, including nearby public transportation routes. In many communities, information on nearby parking is useful.
- **Office Hours**
  List your office hours and days. If the office staff hours are different or vary, suggest when calls can be made to the business office. In this section, indicate your policy about house calls, evening, weekend, and holiday coverage, if appropriate.
- **Telephone Procedures**

  - State how new clients should make, cancel, or change appointments. Remind patients about canceling appointments as far in advance as possible and mention the circumstances under which you charge for missed appointments. Urge patients to be on time—neither too early nor late.
  - In case of an emergency, patients need to know how to reach you. Explain the answering service arrangements for your practice. Describe your procedures for returning phone calls to clients (at the end of each hour, during specific times each day, at the end of the day, etc.). Explanation of answering procedures is calming and can also discourage nonemergency, after-hours calls.
  - If there is a best time to phone for appointments—usually when the receptionist is available or when the schedule is likely to be light—note those

times and encourage patients to call during those hours. List any special telephone numbers or extensions for insurance- and billing-related inquiries.

■ **Fees, Billing, and Collection System**

- Tell clients about your fees; generally stating that care is taken to establish fees that are competitive with other practices in the area is sufficient. It is not, however, necessary or desirable to list fees for specific treatments.
- State that payment is due at the time of service if that is your policy. Indicate whether you handle insurance billing for clients or supply them with the information needed to file their own claims. If you will arrange payment plans for large bills, be sure to mention it in the brochure.
- State the major insurance programs in which you participate: Blue Shield, Medicare, Medicaid, HMOs, and PPOs (by name).

■ **Records**

- Assure patients that no information will be released by your office to insurance companies, attorneys, or others without their written consent.
- If you charge for filling out statements for attorneys or for appearing in court, you might note your policy.

How to Prepare a Client Information Brochure

- Begin with a paragraph that welcomes clients to your practice. Describe the image you wish to project.
- Write in a friendly, personal, and conversational tone; avoid an authoritarian approach even when you feel strongly about a topic. Explain your policies, when possible, in terms of the client's self-interest.
- Work with a reputable graphic designer and printer to help you decide on format, typeface, and method of reproduction. Have your booklet printed in an easy-to-read 10- to 12-point typeface on a durable, light-colored paper.
- Consider using the graphic designer to create a professional-looking logo for your practice and use this logo as part of the design for your booklet. If appropriate for your practice, you might consider having your booklet translated into another language.
- Initially, order what you estimate to be a 6-month supply of booklets. You will probably want to make frequent revisions to the early editions.

The brochure should be tailored to your individual personality, type of practice, and office staff. What is important is to thoroughly and thoughtfully describe your practice policies.

Through good communications you can establish an improved relationship with your clients and enjoy the benefits of a smooth-running practice. Your staff will appreciate having a tool to help inform and educate patients. And your patients will be pleased not only with their therapy and treatment but with your thoughtfulness and management.

Outline for a Proposal to a Managed Care Organization

Elements that might be included in a proposal to a managed care organization (MCO) are useful in other proposals as well. To determine which elements should be included, consider what the client needs and how you can best present your practice as the service provider.

Before you make any proposal, however, investigate the MCO thoroughly to make sure that it is one you wish to join and serve. Find out about their administrative procedures and UR requirements from others who are panel members. Ask yourself some basic questions about the possible relationship between your practice and the MCO.

- How many new patients is this MCO likely to bring to my practice?
- What burdens will joining another MCO place on my office staff?
- What types of records will I have to keep? Are they different from those I keep now?
- Will I have to change my office hours or appointment schedule to accommodate the new patients?
- How much income will this contract bring into the practice?
- What will cash flow look like based on the proposed payment method (if you find out in advance how payment will be made)?
- How do other psychologists who are members of the MCO's panel rate it in terms of clinical standards, administrative hassles, and business relationships?

When you have satisfied yourself that this proposal should be written, follow this general outline:

- **Letter of transmittal.** One-page letter indicating that the practice is pleased to submit this proposal (either as requested or unsolicited) to provide services for the MCO.
- **Cover or title page.** Use special report covers with logo (if available). Cover text is simple: Proposal to The MCO/Client, submitted by The Practice, date of submission, and, if the proposal is in response to a formal request, the request number or identification.
- **Abstract or summary (optional).** If the proposal is longer than eight pages, a summary is helpful.
- **Table of contents (optional).** Use only if the proposal is longer than eight pages.
- **Introduction.** A general statement of why this proposal is needed at this time. You can often recap the local market environment, changes in the delivery of mental health services, general need for mental health services (statistics about mental health needs of the general population, lost work time due to stress, effects of layoffs on workforce, etc.). Condense the introduction into one or two paragraphs.
- **Needs assessment.** Describe what you know about the potential client and their need for mental health services. For example, you can obtain information

from the MCO or the state insurance commissioner's office about the size of the MCO, its operations in the past, which employers it services, and so forth.

If your proposal is in response to a request, the request form will indicate the services that are to be addressed. It is still a good idea to let the client know that you have researched their situation by including MCO-specific data in this section.

- **Practice products and services.** Describe what your practice can offer in resolving the client's problem or filling his or her general mental health needs. If you are offering several services, consider summarizing them in this section of the proposal and appending a one-page (or less) description of each. This section might also include information on

  - How the client would access your services; how your office is organized to handle patient identification and questions about coverage
  - The relationship between you and the client (formal contract with inclusion on provider panel, verbal agreement that you are included in their referral list, etc.)
  - What information or reports you would provide to the client about utilization and a schedule for preparing and submitting the reports
  - Record-keeping systems
  - How the services will be administered at the practice
  - Who (by job title) will perform the services.

  Put yourself in the client's role and think of all of the questions you would ask. Include all the answers in this proposal or be prepared to answer them during an interview. Remember, the proposal remains with the potential client after your interview is concluded. Make sure that it covers all of the important points.

- **Evaluation.** Discuss how you and the client will judge the success of this relationship. This might include number of patients referred, average length of treatment, patient satisfaction, and so on. Include in this section a description (in lay terms) of your usual measurements of success.
- **Capabilities statement.** This document can be separate from the proposal or integrated into the text. It should answer one basic question: "Why is your practice the ideal service to solve the client's problems?" Systems to measure efficiency and effectiveness are particularly important to MCOs.
- **Pricing and budget.** Depending on the type of service that you are proposing, draw up a price list per service or a project budget. In some cases, you may want to indicate that the rates quoted are valid for a limited period of time, perhaps 90 days from the date of submission. Some requests for proposals will ask that all financial information be submitted in a separate document. If that is not requested, include it with the body of the proposal.

  You probably will not be able to determine whether your services are less costly than other practitioners in the community. Stress the procedures in your office that keep costs in line (computerization of the intake process, electronic record keeping and claims filing, review of overhead on a quarterly basis, establishment of practice guidelines that are based on both clinical effectiveness and cost, etc.).

- **Timetable or work plan (if applicable).**
- **Organization chart (if applicable).**
- **Appendix.** Résumés of key staff are frequently appended to proposals. You may have other promotional materials that could be included (examples of workshops that you have presented, articles you have written, client brochures, etc.).

Unless otherwise directed, make an appointment with the MCO to present this proposal in person and answer any questions that the client has about your services. Keep that meeting short—if you cannot present your case in 20 minutes, work on it until you can. Leave the proposal with the client and remind yourself to follow up with a telephone call within a week or as indicated by the potential client.

Choosing and Using Consultants

Consultants to Consider

- Accountant
- Attorney
- Banker
- Computer or management information systems expert
- Insurance counselor
- Insurance broker or salesperson
- Management consultant
- Marketing consultant
- Medical management firm
- Real estate broker

When to Use Consultants

- **For practice management functions.**

  - Setting up a new practice or office
  - Financial planning
  - Preparation for audits
  - Systems revision or improvement
  - Embarking on a new venture that requires legal or financial advice
  - Management problems that arise

- **For formation of an alliance, group practice, partnership, or corporation.**

  - Advice on legal structure and the documentation required
  - Accounting advice

- **For personal financial planning.**

How to Choose an Advisor

- **Develop a pool of prospects by checking with**

  - Colleagues who have sought help from consultants or advisors
  - State or local psychological association
  - Friends and associates in other types of businesses
  - Local bar association
  - Local certified public accountant society
  - Associations of professional business consultants

Some Tips on Selecting and Working With Consultants

- Interview several candidates before making the final selection of a consultant or advisor. Determine whether the consultant is experienced in dealing with health care clients in general and, for some engagements, with mental health services in particular. Whenever possible, select someone who is conveniently located. You will be expected to pay all travel expenses, so select someone close by whenever possible.

- Obtain recent references from the consultant's clients who had needs similar to yours or who are involved in mental health. You may want to ask each consultant to give you the name of at least one person who may be critical of his or her work.

- Define your request for the consultant as clearly as possible. If you cannot be specific about your needs, you can waste time and money when the consultant helps you define why he or she is needed.

- Match the qualifications of the consultant with your problem. Not every consultant has experience in every type of problem that practices face. Be wary of any consulting group that claims they can do all types of consulting equally well. Nearly all have specialties and a few weaknesses.

- Do not select a consultant with whom you are not personally compatible. Make sure that his or her philosophy fits with yours. Does his or her philosophy correlate with yours (conservative vs. risky) and is he or she sensitive to your level of business expertise?

- Be sure that the consultant's availability fits with your timetable. Once you have established the timetable, hold the consultant to it.

- Establish the fee and method of computing it before the engagement begins. Consultants have different methods of determining their fees on the basis of the type and length of engagement: flat fee plus direct expenses, hourly rate and expenses, monthly retainer, and so forth. Evaluate whether the complexity of the problem and the length of the proposed engagement requires a contract.

- Do your homework before you meet with a consultant. Gather all of the data that you think a consultant might need. A good start would be to complete the PATs in the Appendix and, if other practices are involved in the consultation, have them complete the PATs too.

- Avoid using the consultant as a group facilitator. If you are working with a group of therapists, be sure that you all agree on what you are requesting from the consultant. This is another way of saying, "do your homework." If you are trying to form a group and the potential members of the group still disagree on its purpose, it is too early to call in a consultant. Keep working together until you are unified. It will save you time and money.

- Assign one person to be the contact for the consultant so that time (and money) is not wasted in working with multiple sources of information.

- Do as much work as possible over the telephone, using conference calls to cut down on travel expenses and therapists' time away from clients.

- Stay in control of the engagement with the consultant. A consultant can help you to develop alternative answers to a problem and offer options for consideration, but the consultant should never be allowed to make the choice. The therapist or practice must commit to action by choosing the best solutions.

- Require that the consultant document the work done for you or the group. Regular, written progress reports, an update of any changes in the schedule, as well as a final report with recommendations, should be minimal requirements.

7

Conclusion

The Practice of the Future

This Guidebook was developed to aid practitioners in taking steps to ensure their survival. Although no single "plan" exists, there are principles and tools, resources and models, and ideas and information that can be applied wherever and however you choose to practice.

Today's mental health practitioners must learn to apply standard business principles to their practices without sacrificing their clinical or ethical integrity. Responses to the problems in the health care delivery system, the influence of MCOs and their practices, and the increased interest of employers in health matters have a direct impact on mental health practices. As the growth of managed care reduces the number of private-pay patients in the market, providers must compete for those who remain. MCOs and employers are establishing rules that providers must follow if they choose to see the patients covered by their programs. The move toward organizing networks of providers will make it more difficult to maintain a solo practice in the new market.

These forces all have an impact on the long-range plans of providers of psychological services. The marketplace is reshaping mental health delivery systems, financing arrangements, and traditional practice patterns. Buyers are seeking providers who understand their interests, operate as they do, and can give assurances that they are providing high-quality services at a competitive cost. Psychologists must consider how their practices will fare in this new environment.

And although the structure of this new environment is not yet clear, the corporatization of health care has a profound effect on the way psychological practices are organized. The successful psychological practice of the future will most likely be larger, more efficient, more business-oriented while still quality conscious, better connected to the therapeutic and medical communities, and more vertically and horizontally integrated than the practice of today.

As it becomes crucial for psychologists to conform their practices to these emerging norms, traditional practice models may no longer be competitive. The continued development of new models (PPOs, IPAs, PHOs) and complex legal entities (professional corporations and limited liability companies) offer the practitioner a wide range of possible practice models. Each of these models has advantages and disadvantages. Legal, personal, financial, and clinical considerations must be taken into account when deciding which of the many possible models for delivery is appropriate. But it is important to remember that no model will meet all of the requirements of every practitioner.

Increasingly, providers and employers are contracting directly with one another. Direct contracting offers employers and providers the opportunity to stream-line health care service delivery, eliminate unnecessary bureaucracy, ensure quality care, and still control costs. When properly executed, direct contracts benefit patients, payers, and providers alike.

Above all, psychologists need to acquire more expertise in the art of doing business. However, the twin goals of thriving professionally and practicing compassionately need not conflict. Remaining competitive will demand that today's practitioner become acquainted with the skills and knowledge needed to run a successful business. Administration, finance, insurance claims filing, communications, personnel, computers, quality improvement and marketing are all sufficiently important to warrant attention by those directing a practice. Good business practices will support and maintain your ability to practice in an ethical, professional way.

Striving professionally means having a well-run office. And the offices themselves should be warm and inviting, as well as professional and easily accessible. Striving professionally means being responsive to new clients and offering flexible scheduling. A successful practice will always appear fully and professionally staffed and will manage the time of its employees well. It will have excellent communications systems that help it run smoothly. Maintaining complete business records and managing relations with third-party payers will be a matter of routine, along with maintaining a detailed but separate clinical record.

Good financial practices are just as important as good administrative practices. Providers need to become familiar with systems that allow them to track various sources of income, expenses, the impact of new contracts, and the effectiveness of marketing efforts. Developing clearly defined billing policies and procedures, and relating these policies to clients, is an essential part of good financial management. A regular review of a practice's fiscal state is also essential to long-range planning and financial stability.

Adopting the latest computer and management information systems technology can bring greater efficiency and quality improvement even to a small practice. Clinical and business records, billing, claims submissions, scheduling, outcome data collection, interoffice and out-of-office communications, and collection of utilization data can all be made far easier, faster, and more accurate by automating systems.

Successful practices will embrace the idea that continually improving and monitoring quality is an essential function. Quality may be assessed in terms of client satisfaction, clinical outcomes, cost effectiveness, value, and so on. At the local level, practice guidelines and clinical protocols will be developed in the interests of matching patients with the most effective, efficient treatments and providers. Psychologists, whose training in research and data collection methodologies is unparalleled, can easily have a competitive edge in this area.

Finally, marketing is the key to fulfilling the goals of a practice. Although strategies for marketing are many and varied, the targets are simple: new patients, referral sources, and large purchasers. To market effectively it is necessary to find out what these customers need and want and then demonstrate that you can fulfill that need. Tracking the quality and value of a practice is essential to effective marketing efforts.

With this Guidebook we have endeavored to give you many of the tools and much of the knowledge that you will need to succeed in today's market. It will serve you best as a reference and a guide to help you ask the right questions and know when to seek the help of a consultant. This is, of course, meant to be a document that is revised and updated as often as developments in the field of mental health warrant. Toward that aim we encourage you to provide feedback on both its content and presentation. As providers, you are the ultimate test of what works and what does not. And ultimately, it is your initiative, courage, and dedication that will ensure your future success and the future success of psychology.

Appendix

Practice Analysis Tools
American Psychological Association Resources
Record Keeping Guidelines

Practice Analysis Tools

Listed below are the Practice Analysis Tools contained in this Appendix. A brief purpose for each tool is included here; more detailed suggestions for use are listed as each tool is presented in the text. Although all of the tools should be helpful to most practices, some may not seem appropriate for solo practices, small groups, or partnerships. Review each tool before answering the questions or filling in the blanks. Involve your staff in completing the forms so that all the participants in the practice share the same view.

Title	Page	Purpose
Practice Record	120	Summary of practice; use in proposals, capability statements, brochures, letter of petition to a managed care organization, and so on
Staff and Services	122	Categorization of staff capabilities and areas of specialization; use in capability statements and strategic and human resources planning
Area Market Data	124	Recap of community; use in strategic planning, marketing, comparison of practice statistics with community statistics to determine degree of match
Referral Base	127	Analysis of how patients reach your practice; crucial data for marketing; identifies referral patterns and gaps, suggests natural alliances with other practitioners, and tracks results of marketing activity
Patient–Payer Profile	130	Record of income sources; use in financial planning; identifies overreliance on single payer, suggests untapped revenue sources, and indicates possible geographical areas that are not covered
Business Management	133	Review of business practices; record of operations; basics for strategic planning
Quality Improvement	136	Record of treatment profiles; gives overview of patient mix; sets the stage for quality improvement

Practice Record

The following easy-to-complete, one-page record is a snapshot of your practice. You can use it to

- Develop a statement of the capabilities of the practice that might accompany a proposal
- Introduce your services to potential new clients
- Form the basis for a petition to an HMO
- Start off a brochure about the practice that could be distributed to potential referrers.

Tips for the Practitioner:

- Update your Practice Record annually after you have conducted a full practice review (using all of the forms in this section) and revised your strategic plan for the year.

- If your practice is changing rapidly, update more frequently. Never let the information about your practice become so outdated that you cannot respond quickly to potential target markets.

Practice Record Form

Name of the practice _____

Number of years in operation _____

Predominant type of practice   _____ Solo

                       _____ Single specialty group

                       _____ Multidisciplinary group

                       _____ Office sharing (solo practitioners sharing office expenses but not profits)

                       _____ Hospital-based group

                       _____ Academic medical group

                       _____ Other

Number of credentialed practitioners in the practice _____

     Number of practitioners with MD _____

     Number of practitioners with PhD _____

     Number of practitioners with MSW _____

Number of other employees in the practice by category

     Clerical   _____

     Administrative or management   _____

     Other (specify job titles)   _____   _____

                                             _____

Total number of clients treated in your practice in the past year _____

List each program, product, or service that you provide. If these services have been accredited, cite the accrediting body (Council on Accreditation of Rehabilitation Facilities, Council of Behavioral Group Practices, American Board of Certified Managed Care Providers, etc.).

_____

_____

_____

Describe the goals of your practice or list your mission statement.

_____

_____

_____

_____

_____

_____

_____

_____

Staff and Services

The following Fact Sheet captures the credentialing, licensing, and educational information about each of the principals, therapists, and counselors in your practice. In addition, their areas of service, personal interest, and patient services are indicated, along with their personal treatment preferences. Each staff member should complete a Fact Sheet and update the data on a regular basis.

On a separate page, write a paragraph describing each of these services. The descriptions should be free of jargon, note the types of patients (or condition) that are covered by the service, and note the results of using the service.

Combining the data from all of the staff Fact Sheets

- recaps the strengths of the staff
- identifies whether there are specialty areas that are not covered (or desired)
- the descriptions of services might be used in proposals, capability statements, brochures, and other literature about your practice
- helps plan for human resources, space, and equipment needs.

A review of the Staff and Services forms may answer questions about the need to add additional therapists in order to give depth to the practice, what support staff might be used to deal with group activities, and whether there is sufficient space and equipment for all of the staff to operate efficiently.

Tips for the Practitioner:

- Review and update this information every 6 months. Ask each staff member to complete his or her own Fact Sheet and help with writing the program descriptions.
- Ask someone who is not in the mental health field to read your program descriptions to ensure they are jargon-free and easy to understand.
- If necessary, hire an editor to pare down your service descriptions to concise, clear statements.

Fact Sheet

Name: Gender: Age:

Education/advanced degrees/licenses:

Additional credentials or citations:

Local/regional/national institutes, universities, or organizations to which you belong and positions you hold:

Describe the specific treatment philosophy or philosophies to which you subscribe:

Check the areas of service you provide, rank them in the order of time spent, and indicate those areas in which you specialize or would like to specialize.

Areas of Service	Rank by Time Spent	Specialization (current or future)
Adult mental health	_____	_____
Child mental health	_____	_____
Adolescent mental health	_____	_____
Adult substance abuse	_____	_____
Child or adolescent substance abuse	_____	_____
Disability or handicap evaluation	_____	_____
Survivors of childhood abuse	_____	_____
Survivors of sexual abuse	_____	_____
Survivors of trauma	_____	_____
Couples/marital	_____	_____
Eating disorders	_____	_____
Other (specify)	_____	_____

Check the types of patient services you provide, rank them in order of time spent, and check those that represent your personal preferences.

Patient Services	Rank by Time Spent	Personal Preference
Individual therapy	_____	_____
Group therapy	_____	_____
Marriage and family therapy	_____	_____
Behavioral therapy	_____	_____
Cognitive therapy	_____	_____
Pain management	_____	_____
Psychological testing	_____	_____
Neuropsychological assessment	_____	_____
Biofeedback	_____	_____
Disability evaluation	_____	_____
Other (specify)	_____	_____

Area Market Data

This section will help you to identify the factors in the local market that affect the need for your services. This section characterizes the community in ways that will direct your marketing efforts to specific targets, identify some of your competitors, and corroborate trends in mental health care so that you may anticipate changes that will affect your practice.

Although you will be tempted to answer most of the questions by guessing, finding the real answers may lead to new insights. Call your local library or state or city economic development office to obtain census data. Also ask them for sources for the managed care data. Local hospitals often have collected what you need to know about the community. Ask for the planning department—they are usually quite willing to share their information.

Tips for the Practitioner:

- Make someone in the practice responsible for compiling market updates. Clip articles from the local papers, review appropriate periodicals that deal with managed care and insurance developments, and scan professional journals for new practice ideas.
- If you are in a large metropolitan area, find out if any organizations track demographics by neighborhood or zip codes (mailing list distributors, local newspapers, civic organizations).
- Get on the mailing list of the local business and health coalition if one exists in your community.
- As you plan for the future of your practice, keep reminding yourself of the predictable changes in your community (aging of the population as a whole, shifts in ages of residents in particular areas).

Area Market Data Form

Describe the market in which your main practice or office is located.

_____ Total city and suburban population, 1 million or more
_____ Total city and suburban population, 500,000 to 999,999
_____ Total city and suburban population, 100,000 to 499,999
_____ Under 100,000

Is the population

_____ growing
_____ stable
_____ declining

What percentage of the population in your market is 65 years of age or older?

_____ %

What percentage of the population in your market is under 21 years of age?

_____ %

Is your market dominated by one or a few large employers?

_____ Yes
_____ No

List the prominent employers in your community and indicate whether they have an EAP.

	EAP?
_____	_____
_____	_____
_____	_____
_____	_____
_____	_____
_____	_____
_____	_____
_____	_____
_____	_____

Estimate the percentage of the total population in your market whose mental health care is provided by an MCO. (Total population should include the uninsured and unemployed, as well as those covered by Medicare and Medicaid.)

_____ 0%–10%
_____ 11%–40%
_____ 41% or more
_____ Don't know

(Continued on next page)

(Area Market Data continued)

List the five largest or most successful MCOs in your community that offer mental health benefits.

_____

_____

_____

_____

_____

Describe any other market factors that affect psychologists and their practices. Consider whether you must compete with large and active public health clinics or university practices and be concerned about your community's unemployment rates, the average family income and educational levels, predominant race and ethnic groups and their attitudes toward mental health services, and so forth.

_____

_____

_____

_____

_____

_____

Referral Base

Keeping track of how patients reach your practice provides vital data for your marketing program. If most of your patients are self-referrals or referrals from other clients, you may want to find ways to enhance those sources: continued contact with patients after conclusion of therapy through newsletters, periodic personal notes, and distribution of relevant articles. If your sources are primarily from other psychologists, make sure you contact them frequently. Practitioners often refer to those counselors whom they saw most recently.

If you have placed advertisements or announcements in local media, be sure to record which announcements got results.

For the future, make sure your computer software can record how each new patient selected you—no more searching through the records by hand when you want to look at your referral base. Let the computer do it for you.

Tips for the Practitioner:

- Collect the data about referrals at the same time you complete the patient profile. That way you will need to review files only once to obtain all of the information you need.
- Review your overall referral patterns. Is more than 20% of your total patient load or revenue from a single source? If so, you should do everything you can to ensure that that source will not dwindle. Or establish a marketing plan that will build the contribution of other sources.

Referral Data Form

Referral source	Number of Patients	Percentage of Patients
Individuals		
Self	_____	_____
Another patient or client	_____	_____
Other psychologists	_____	_____
Physicians	_____	_____
Other professionals	_____	_____
Pharmacists	_____	_____
Social workers	_____	_____
Nurses	_____	_____
Clergy	_____	_____
Other	_____	_____
Businesses		
Insurance companies	_____	_____
EAPs	_____	_____
Employers	_____	_____
Others	_____	_____
Health Care Organizations		
Hospitals		
Emergency room activities	_____	_____
Nonphysician staff	_____	_____
Formal referral service	_____	_____
MCOs		
HMO (name) _____	_____	_____
PPO (name) _____	_____	_____
Other (name) _____	_____	_____
Other Activities of Therapists in the Practice		
Teaching activities	_____	_____
Community activities	_____	_____
Speeches or articles	_____	_____
Social contacts (list):	_____	_____
Advertising		
Yellow Pages	_____	_____
Radio	_____	_____
TV	_____	_____
Newspaper (community)	_____	_____
Distribution of practice brochure	_____	_____
Professional association listing	_____	_____
Welcome Wagon or newcomers' services	_____	_____

Referral Data Summary:

How do your patients find out about you?

_____ %   self-referral
_____ %   another patient/client
_____ %   other psychologists
_____ %   physicians
_____ %   other health professionals
_____ %   businesses (including EAPs)
_____ %   health care organizations
        _____ % HMOs (list each) _____
                         _____
                         _____

        _____ % PPOs (list each) _____
                         _____
                         _____

_____ %   direct marketing (direct mail, meeting with groups, giving workshops or speeches)
_____ %   all other

Patient–Payer Profile

Much of the information discussed in this section can be captured using the following form (note items marked with an asterisk). Organizing all of the data about patients and payers (plus some community information) helps in putting the pieces together.
Review the ages of the patients that you served during the past year.

■ Compare the percentages with the information you have about the age distribution in the total population. Do you serve some groups more often or better than others? Are your services deliberately geared to a particular age group?

■ Are there some age categories that you are not serving? These data could help you develop a marketing plan aimed either at increasing the number of patients in the age group you serve well or obtaining new patients in a different age group.

One of the most important factors in financial planning is determining where your payments are coming from at the present time. If you have the data, compare the payer profile for the last 3 years to determine whether the base is shifting from one payer to another. Check the profile to see whether you are relying too heavily on one or a few payers. What would happen if those payers decided to contract with someone else? Would it have a small or devastating effect on your practice? If the answer is devastating, start looking for patients that will give you a more balanced payer base.

Tips for the Practitioner:

- Have a diverse number of financial classes in your payer base.
- Become experienced in fee-for-service reimbursement before taking a capitated contract.
- If you determine you *must* change your payer base in order to stay in business but are unsure how to do it, get professional marketing consultation.
- Do not take on several new contracts at the same time. Try to phase them in a few months apart so that you can become thoroughly familiar with each before moving to another.

Patient–Payer Profile Form

What percentage of your active patients are
_____ 65 years of age or over
_____ aged 56–65
_____ aged 21–45
_____ aged 13–20
_____ under age 13
100% total

Where do your patients reside? Tabulate by zip code.*
Where do your patients work? Tabulate by zip code.*
If known, tabulate ethnic or cultural information about your patients that might be meaningful in your community.*

What percentage of your practice revenue is derived from each of the following? Are these sources of revenue decreasing, increasing, or remaining stable?

Revenue source	Decreasing	Stable	Increasing
_____% Medicaid	☐	☐	☐
_____% Medicare	☐	☐	☐
_____% Managed care (HMOs and PPOs)	☐	☐	☐
_____% Self-pay	☐	☐	☐
_____% Commercial insurance companies	☐	☐	☐
_____% Blue Cross and Blue Shield	☐	☐	☐
Is your pro bono work	☐	☐	☐

What is the total number of contracts your practice has with managed care organizations? (Include HMOs, PPOs, POS, and direct contracting.)

_____ Number of contracts

How has the payer mix changed in the past 3 years? _____
_____
_____
_____

From a business perspective, how satisfied are you with your current payer mix?
_____
_____
_____
_____

(Continued on next page)

(Patient–Payer Profile continued)

How does the payer mix affect your satisfaction with the practice? For example, are there some payers that you find easy to work with and others that impede your work?

_____

_____

_____

How would you like the payer mix to change in the next 3 years?

_____

_____

_____

_____

In which of the following ways are you and your practice reimbursed? (Check all that apply.)
_____ Fee for service
_____ Discounted fee for service
_____ Discounted fee for service with withhold arrangement
_____ Fee schedule
_____ Fee schedule with withhold arrangement
_____ Global fee
_____ Global fee with stop loss
_____ Capitation
_____ Other (specify)

Are most mental health facilities (clinics, public health service, hospitals, etc.) in your market
_____ Aggressively pursuing managed care contracts
_____ Not very interested in managed care contracts
_____ Aggressively avoiding managed care contracts
_____ Don't know

How will the plans of these facilities affect your practice? _____

_____

_____

_____

Business Management

Practices do not grow or flourish without careful planning and hard work. These business management questions provide you with basic data about the operation of your practice and give you ways to compare performance from one year to another. Review the Financial Practices section in chapter 5 for more details on managing the finances of your practice.

- Do you have a written, long-range strategic plan for your practice?
- Have you established an annual budget for the practice? Yes _____ No _____
     Do you compare actual income and expense to the budget at least every quarter? Yes _____ No _____

Review your accounts receivable. Calculate the average length of time it takes to collect your charges. If most of your bills are collected (from insurance companies as well as private-pay patients) within 60–90 days, your collection procedures are ade-

Collection Period Example
Annual billings: $80,000
Average accounts receivable: $9,310
$\dfrac{9310 \times 365 \text{ days}}{\$80,000} = 42.48 \text{ days}$

quate. But a 45-day collection period would produce a healthier cash flow. Review your collection policies to see whether they could be more aggressive and assure yourself that the policies are being carried out as you designed them.

Another more common measure of collection efficiency is the collection ratio. Calculate by dividing the total collections for the year by the total charges for the year. The result is the percentage of charges that you are able to collect. Collection ratios may range from 80% to 95% or more depending on your source of income and the affluence of your patients. If your practice has less than a 90% collection ra-

Collection Ratio
Collections for current month: $6,400
Collections for previous   11 months: $71,000
Charges for current month: $7,150
Charges for previous 11 months: $76,400
$\dfrac{\$6,400 + \$71,000}{\$7,150 + \$76,400} = \dfrac{\$77,400}{\$83,550} = 92.6\%$

tio, look carefully at which patients or insurance companies are not paying their full bills and adjust your policies and collection procedures for those groups.

- What are your overhead rates, that is, the percentage of gross income that is spent on all office and business expenses except psychologist's income? (Overhead = business expenses/gross income.)
     _____ %

If your practice is conducted in a spacious, high-rent office building and you have a number of support staff working with you, your overhead costs may run as high as 50% of your income. If you are practicing in a home office with no staff, overhead should be very low—perhaps 15% to 20% of income. Whatever the figure, check to see whether you can reduce the overhead without reducing the quality of your services. Do some comparison shopping for the supplies that you buy. Check your staffing levels. Would two part-time employees to whom you pay minimal benefits suit your practice better than one full-time employee with full benefits? Would spending some money—to buy a computer, for example—ultimately reduce your overhead by increasing efficiency?

■ Do you employ support staff? _____ Yes _____ No
   If yes, do you have written job descriptions for each position?
   _____ Yes _____ No
   Does your practice have written employment policies? Do you update them annually? (For example, in 1992 the handbook should have been amended to reflect the passage of legislation affecting the employment of persons with disabilities and the granting of family leave.)
■ Does your practice have written policies regarding the following office operations?

Operation	Yes	No	Planned
Reception area procedures			
Telephone answering protocol			
Telephone message handling			
Scheduling office appointments			
Release of patient information			
Billing procedures			
Collection procedures			
Insurance claims procedures			

■ Does your practice use computers? _____ Yes _____ No
• If yes, do you have an electronic billing program? _____ Yes _____ No
   If no, are your insurance claims filed within 3 days of the patient visit?
   _____ Yes _____ No
• Do you have the ability to collect and arrange data to conduct outcome studies?
• Do you maintain client treatment records electronically?
■ Patient records
• Are they kept in a safe, restricted area so that patient confidentiality is assured?
   _____ yes _____ no
• If computerized, are the records backed up on a regular basis?
   _____ yes _____ no
• Are records current? That is, are progress notes added no later than 48 hours after patient contact?
   _____ yes _____ no

- Are telephone conversations with the patient entered into the record?
  _____ yes _____ no
- Are contacts with MCOs documented?
  _____ yes _____ no
- Are test results recorded?
  _____ yes _____ no
- When a patient fails to show for a scheduled appointment, is it documented in the record? _____ yes _____ no
  Do you follow-up to determine the reason for the cancellation, and is that information recorded? _____ yes _____ no

Listed below are some of the management and administrative skills that you may find necessary to develop effective strategies for enlarging your practice, merging with other practices, or negotiating contracts with MCOs or employers. Which of these skills do you possess? Which skills are adequately covered by other members of your staff? For which would you choose to use a consultant?

Strategic planning: Assessing the market and mental health care environment, establishing goals and objectives for the practice, and identifying specific tasks to achieve those objectives.

☐ Have these skills   ☐ Other staff have these skills   ☐ Will use consultant

Budgeting: Developing an annual budget for the practice and creating the tracking systems needed to assess adherence to the budget.

☐ Have these skills   ☐ Other staff have these skills   ☐ Will use consultant

Evaluating organizations and presenting your practice to specific MCOs, employers, or other groups in order to increase the practice income.

☐ Have these skills   ☐ Other staff have these skills   ☐ Will use consultant

Negotiating contracts with such organizations to your advantage.

☐ Have these skills   ☐ Other staff have these skills   ☐ Will use consultant

Measuring patient satisfaction: Developing surveys, interview protocol, and other devices to determine the patient's or consumer's image of the practice.

☐ Have these skills   ☐ Other staff have these skills   ☐ Will use consultant

Using other experts: Identifying problems that require outside assistance and selecting and directing consultants and other professional services.

☐ Have these skills   ☐ Other staff have these skills

Plans for your own training and education, helping your staff to attain new skills, and the hiring of consultants for special tasks should be part of your budget process.

Quality Improvement

Perhaps the most important data that you can collect about your practice to improve your practice is in this section. Monitoring the details of the types of patients you have treated, the average length of treatment, and success ratios provides you with an excellent view of your professional status. Furthermore, the data can be useful in "selling" your services to MCOs or other providers.

You may want to add questions that are particularly appropriate to the types of cases that you handle so that you can track the improvement in your management of those cases over time.

Tips for the Practitioner:

- If you have never conducted a patient or referrer satisfaction survey in the past, begin now. You could choose to survey patients who completed their therapy in the past 6 months or work with current patients.
- Begin developing practice guidelines by trying the easy ones first. Administrative routines might be the place to start.
- Research everything that you can find on clinical protocols that have been developed by other practices. Begin your practice protocols by adapting what has already been done. Computer access to some large databases—or even some of the computer-user bulletin boards—could be helpful.

Quality Improvement Data

Do you measure your customers' satisfaction levels? _____ Yes _____ No
    If yes, how often do you measure? _____
    What method do you use?
    _____   Written survey
    _____   Survey by phone
    _____   Formal interview/review/conversation
    _____   Informal conversation
    _____   Intuition

    What percentage were satisfied with each of the following practice factors?
        Therapy
            Relationship with the therapist _____ %
            Progress in therapy _____ %
            Outcomes _____ %

        Administration of the practice
            Scheduling _____ %
            Billing _____ %
            Collections _____ %

        Practice amenities _____ %

    If you do analyze satisfaction levels, do you include both current and past patients?
    _____ Yes _____ No

Do you measure the satisfaction of those professionals who refer patients to you?
    _____ Yes _____ No

    If yes, are they satisfied with the speed with which you see their referrals?
    _____ Yes _____ No

    Are they satisfied with the reports that you provided about the care of their patient?
    _____ Yes _____ No

Are they satisfied with the quality of care you provided?
    _____ Yes _____ No

Has your practice developed or adopted written practice guidelines?
    _____ Yes _____ No

    If yes, do these guidelines include (check all that apply)
    _____   Administrative procedures regarding clinical information flow,
                follow-up and documentation
    _____   Directions for developing treatment plans
    _____   Referral indicators and procedures
    _____   Clinical management of specific conditions
    _____   Other

(Continued on next page)

(*Quality Improvement continued*)

Has your practice developed or adopted quality measurements?
_____ Yes   _____ No
If yes, do these measurements include (check all that apply)
_____   Definition of therapeutic success
_____   Rate of therapeutic success
_____   Protocols for intake interviews
_____   Peer review mechanisms (internal or with professionals from
             other practices)
_____   Follow-up procedures on referrals to determine appropriateness

List at least two aspects of your practice that reflect innovation. They may be related to practice areas or techniques, an internal peer review system, or the configuration of your office space. What sets you apart from other practitioners?

_____
_____
_____
_____
_____

Distribution of Patients by Diagnosis

Listed below are types of problems or diagnoses that you may treat. Indicate the average number of visits each diagnostic group typically requires. Collect this information on each practicing psychologist in the practice as well as for the practice as a whole.

Problems or Diagnoses	Number of Patients	Average Number of Visits			
		1–10	11–20	21–50	51 or more
Anxiety disorders					
Phobias					
Dissociative disorders					
Sexual abuse					
Sexual dysfunction					
Physical abuse					
Affective disorders and depression					
Eating disorders					
Marital problems					
Family problems					
Gender issues					
Attention deficit hyperactive disorders					
Posttraumatic stress disorders					
Alcohol and chemical dependency					
Psychotic disorders					
Organic mental disorders					
Education and learning disorders					
Chronic pain					
Personality disorders					
Other					
Other					
Other					
Other					

American Psychological Association Resources

American Psychological Association Insurance Trust.

Comparison of Utilization Review and Benefit Design Approaches to Controlling Outpatient Mental Health Care Costs, APA Practice Directorate. A white paper that reviews the data showing that outpatient utilization review is not as cost-effective as originally hoped and that changes in co-insurance and coverage limits are much more cost-effective.

Computer Use in Psychology: A Directory of Software (3rd ed.), M. L. Stoloff & J. V. Couch, Eds., APA Books, 1992.

The Economics and Effectiveness of Inpatient and Outpatient Mental Health Treatment, APA Practice Directorate. A brief analysis that shows that for several patient populations, outpatient therapy is as effective and significantly more cost-effective than inpatient therapy.

The Effectiveness of Psychological Services in Improving Employee Productivity and Attendance, APA Practice Directorate. An annotated bibliography of studies and journal articles that show that mental illness and substance abuse reduced overall worker productivity while increasing absenteeism, accident proneness, and turnover. Furthermore, the efficacy of psychotherapy in treating the disorders leading to poor work performance is reviewed.

The Efficacy of Psychotherapy, APA Practice Directorate. A review of some of the major studies and articles that demonstrate the efficacy of psychotherapy.

Ethical Principles of Psychologists and Code of Conduct, §§ 1.25, 5.11 concerning fee collection, APA Council of Representatives.

Hardware, Software, and the Mental Health Profession: The Complete Guide to Office Computerization, M. L. Stoloff, J. V. Couch, & J. Brewster, Eds., APA Books, 1991.

The Impact of Integrated Care, APA Practice Directorate. The actual claims data and actuarial projections included in this paper show how businesses can and have reduced mental health costs by adopting the principles of integrated care.

The Medical Cost Offset, APA Practice Directorate. An annotated bibliography of studies that demonstrate that people with mental illness reduce their over-utilization of medical services when receiving adequate mental health care.

The Legal and Legislative Considerations of Prescription Privileges for Psychologists, Office of Legal & Regulatory Affairs, APA Practice Directorate.

The Psychologist's Legal Handbook, Clifford D. Stromberg, Hogan & Hartson, Washington, DC.

Psychotherapy and Depression, APA Practice Directorate. A review of the literature on the prevalence and impact of depression and the effectiveness of psychological intervention in the treatment of depressed patients.

Record Keeping Guidelines, Committee on Professional Practice & Standards of the APA Board of Professional Affairs.

Training in Mental Health Diagnosis and Treatment, APA Practice Directorate. A chart and corresponding bar graph that compare the duration and intensity of education and practice experience among psychologists, psychiatrists, and social workers.

Record Keeping Guidelines

*Drafted by the Committee on Professional Practice &
Standards, A Committee of the
Board of Professional Affairs
Adopted by the Council of Representatives,
February 1993*

Introduction[1]

The guidelines that follow are based on the General Guidelines, adopted by the American Psychological Association (APA) in July 1987 (APA, 1987). The guidelines receive their inspirational guidance from specific APA *Ethical Principles of Psychologists and Code of Conduct* (APA, 1992).

These guidelines are aspirational and professional judgment must be used in specific applications. They are intended for use by providers of health care services.[2,3]

Reprinted from the *American Psychologist*, 48, 984–986. Copyright 1993 by the American Psychological Association.

[1]In 1988 the Board of Professional Affairs (BPA) directed the Committee on Professional Practice and Standards (COPPS) to determine whether record keeping guidelines would be appropriate. COPPS was informed that these guidelines would supplement the provisions contained in the *General Guidelines for Providers of Psychological Services*, which had been amended two years earlier. The Council of Representatives approved the General Guidelines records provisions after extended debate on the minimum recordation concerning the nature and contents of psychological services. The General Guidelines reflect a compromise position that psychologists hold widely varying views on the wisdom of recording the content of the psychotherapeutic relationship. In light of the Council debate on the content of psychological records and the absence of an integrated document, BPA instructed COPPS to assess the need for such guidelines, and, if necessary, the likely content.

COPPS undertook a series of interviews with psychologists experienced in this area. The consensus of the respondents indicated that practicing psychologists could benefit from guidance in this area. In addition, an APA legal intern undertook a 50-state review of laws governing psychologists with respect to record keeping provisions. The survey demonstrated that while some states have relatively clear provisions governing certain types of records, many questions are often left unclear. In addition, there is a great deal of variability among the states, so that consistent treatment of records as people move from state to state, or as records are sought from other states, may not be easy to achieve.

Based on COPPS' survey and legal research, BPA in 1989 directed COPPS to prepare an initial set of record keeping guidelines. This document resulted.

[2]These guidelines apply to Industrial/Organizational psychologists providing health care services but generally not to those providing nonhealth care I/O services. For instance, in I/O psychology, written records may constitute the primary work product, such as a test instrument or a job analysis, while psychologists providing health care services may principally use records to document non-written services and to maintain continuity.

[3]Rather than keeping their own record system, psychologists practicing in institutional settings comply with the institution's policies on record keeping, so long as they are consistent with legal and ethical standards.

143

The language of these guidelines must be interpreted in light of their aspirational intent, advancements in psychology and the technology of record keeping, and the professional judgment of the individual psychologist. It is important to highlight that professional judgment is not preempted by these guidelines: rather, the intent is to enhance it.

Underlying Principles and Purpose

Psychologists maintain records for a variety of reasons, the most important of which is the benefit of the client. Records allow a psychologist to document and review the delivery of psychological services. The nature and extent of the record will vary depending upon the type and purpose of psychological services. Records can provide a history and current status in the event that a user seeks psychological services from another psychologist or mental health professional.

Conscientious record keeping may also benefit psychologists themselves, by guiding them to plan and implement an appropriate course of psychological services, to review work as a whole, and to self-monitor more precisely.

Maintenance of appropriate records may also be relevant for a variety of other institutional, financial, and legal purposes. State and federal laws in many cases require maintenance of appropriate records of certain kinds of psychological services. Adequate records may be a requirement for receipt of third party payment for psychological services.

In addition, well documented records may help protect psychologists from professional liability, if they become the subject of legal or ethical proceedings. In these circumstances, the principal issue will be the professional action of the psychologist, as reflected in part by the records.

At times, there may be conflicts between the federal, state or local laws governing record keeping, the requirements of institutional rules, and these guidelines. In these circumstances, psychologists bear in mind their obligations to conform to applicable law. When laws or institutional rules appear to conflict with the principles of these guidelines, psychologists use their education, skills and training to identify the relevant issues, and to attempt to resolve it in a way that, to the maximum extent feasible, conforms both to law and to professional practice, as required by ethical principles.

Psychologists are justifiably concerned that, at times, record keeping information will be required to be disclosed against the wishes of the psychologist or client, and may be released to persons unqualified to interpret such records. These guidelines assume that no record is free from disclosure all of the time, regardless of the wishes of the client or the psychologist.

1. Content of Records

a. Records include any information (including information stored in a computer) that may be used to document the nature, delivery, progress, or results of psychological services. Records can be reviewed and duplicated.

b. Records of psychological services minimally include (a) identifying data, (b) dates of services, (c) types of services, (d) fees, (e) any assessment, plan for intervention, consultation, summary reports, and/or testing reports and supporting data as may be appropriate, and (f) any release of information obtained.

c. As may be required by their jurisdiction and circumstances, psychologists maintain to a reasonable degree accurate, current, and pertinent records of psychological services. The detail is sufficient to permit planning for continuity in the event that another psychologist takes over delivery of services, including, in the event of death, disability, and retirement. In addition, psychologists maintain records in sufficient detail for regulatory and administrative review of psychological service delivery.

d. Records kept beyond the minimum requirements are a matter of professional judgment for the psychologist. The psychologist takes into account the nature of the psychological services, the source of the information recorded, the intended use of the records, and his or her professional obligation.

e. Psychologists make reasonable efforts to protect against the misuse of records. They take into account the anticipated use by the intended or anticipated recipients when preparing records. Psychologists adequately identify impressions and tentative conclusions as such.

2. Construction and Control of Records

a. Psychologists maintain a system that protects the confidentiality of records. They must take reasonable steps to establish and maintain the confidentiality of information arising from their own delivery of psychological services, or the services provided by others working under their supervision.

b. Psychologists have ultimate responsibility for the content of their records and the records of those under their supervision. Where appropriate, this requires that the psychologist oversee the design and implementation of record keeping procedures, and monitor their observance.

c. Psychologists maintain control over their clients' records, taking into account the policies of the institutions in which they practice. In situations where psychologists have control over their clients' records and where circumstances change such that it is no longer feasible to maintain control over such records, psychologists seek to make appropriate arrangements for transfer.

d. Records are organized in a manner that facilitates their use by the psychologist and other authorized persons. Psychologists strive to assure that record entries are legible. Records are to be completed in a timely manner.

e. Records may be maintained in a variety of media, so long as their utility, confidentiality and durability are assured.

3. Retention of Records

a. The psychologist is aware of relevant federal, state and local laws and regulations governing record retention. Such laws and regulations supersede the requirements of these guidelines. In the absence of such laws and regulations, complete records are maintained for a minimum of 3 years after the last contact with the client. Records, or a summary, are then maintained for an additional 12 years before disposal.[4] If the client is a minor, the record period is extended until 3 years after the age of majority.

b. All records, active and inactive, are maintained safely, with properly limited access, and from which timely retrieval is possible.

4. Outdated Records

a. Psychologists are attentive to situations in which record information has become outdated, and may therefore be invalid, particularly in circumstances where disclosure might cause adverse effects. Psychologists ensure that when disclosing such information that its outdated nature and limited utility are noted using professional judgment and complying with applicable law.

b. When records are to be disposed of, this is done in an appropriate manner that ensures nondisclosure (or preserves confidentiality) (see Section 3a).

5. Disclosure of Record Keeping Procedures

a. When appropriate, psychologists may inform their clients of the nature and extent of their record keeping procedures. This information includes a statement on the limitations of the confidentiality of the records.

b. Psychologists may charge a reasonable fee for review and reproduction of records. Psychologists do not withhold records that are needed for valid healthcare purposes solely because the client has not paid for prior services.

References

American Psychological Association. (1987). General guidelines for providers of psychological services. *American Psychologist, 42*, 712–723.
American Psychological Association. (1992). Ethical principles of psychologists and code of conduct. *American Psychologist, 47*, 1597–1611.

---

[4]These time limits follow the APA's specialty guidelines. If the specialty guidelines should be revised, a simple 7 year requirement for the retention of the complete record is preferred, which would be a more stringent requirement than any existing state statute.

Selected References

Chapter 2   Environmental Assessment: A Look at the Health Care and Mental Health Care Marketplace

American Psychological Association, Practice Directorate. (1992). *Survival guide for the 1990s: A marketing handbook for psychologists*. Washington, DC: Author.

Psychotherapy Finances Staff. (1993). *Managed care handbook*. Jupiter, FL: Ridgewood Financial Institute, Inc.

The state of health care in America [Special issue]. (1993). *Business & Health*.

Stromberg, C. D. (1988). *The psychologist's legal handbook*. Washington, DC: Council for the National Register of Health Service Providers in Psychology.

U.S. Congressional Budget Office. (1993, June). *Trends in health spending: An update*. Washington, DC: U.S. Government Printing Office.

U.S. General Accounting Office. (1993). *Managed care* (Rep. No. GAO/HRD-94-3, B-254303). Washington, DC: U.S. Government Printing Office.

Chapter 3   Trends in Mental Health Care Delivery

Fine, A. (1991, May). Direct purchase contracts carry risks and benefits. *Healthcare Financial Management, 45*, 40–43.

Halbert, L. A. (1988, July–August). Self-insurer's costs can be reduced by direct contracting. *Journal of Compensation and Benefits, 4*, 12–14.

Jones, L. (1993, December 27). Still some hurdles to mental health coverage. *American Medical News*, pp. 1, 5.

Psychiatric care delivery is improving [Special report]. (1993). *Business & Health*.

Putting outcomes research to work [Special report]. (1993). *Business & Health*.

What the experts advise [Special report]. (1991). *Business & Health*.

When a new mental health company got the contract, the established therapists got tossed off the panel. (1992, September). *Managed Care Strategies*, p. 2.

Chapter 4   Models of Practice

American Psychological Association, Office of Managed Care, Legal & Regulatory Affairs. *Memorandum addressed to persons interested in HMO/PPO information*. Washington, DC: Author.

American Psychological Association, Office of Managed Care, Legal & Regulatory Affairs. (1993, August). *State insurance laws affecting preferred provider organizations* (Draft). Washington, DC: Author.

American Psychological Association, Office of Managed Care, Legal & Regulatory Affairs. (1993, December). *State laws affecting health maintenance organizations* (Draft). Washington, DC: Author.

American Psychological Association, Office of Managed Care, Legal & Regulatory Affairs. (1993, August). *State statutes regulating utilization review* (Draft). Washington, DC: Author.

Newman, R. S., & Bricklin, P. (1991). Parameters of managed mental health care: Legal, ethical, and professional guidelines. *Professional Psychology: Research and Practice, 22*, 26–35.

Psychotherapy Finances Staff. (1992). *Managed care handbook*. Jupiter, FL: Ridgewood Financial Institute, Inc.

Stromberg, C. D. (1988). *The psychologist's legal handbook*. Washington, DC: The Council for the National Register of Health Service Providers in Psychology.

Chapter 5   Developing Plans

Shortell, S. M. (1992). *Strategic management of health services organizations*. Boston: Kent Publishing.

Woody, R. H. (1989). *Business success in mental health practice*. San Francisco: Jossey-Bass.

Chapter 6   Successful Business Practices

American Psychological Association. (1992). Ethical principles of psychologists and code of conduct. *American Psychologist, 47*, 1597–1611.

American Psychological Association Practice Directorate and the Ohio Psychological Association. (1985). Marketing psychological services. *Proceedings of the Ohio Psychological Association 1985 Marketing Conference*. Washington, DC: Author.

American Psychological Association, Committee on Professional Practice & Standards. (1993). Record keeping guidelines. *American Psychologist, 48*, 984–986.

Baum, N. (1992). *Marketing your clinical practice: Ethically, effectively, economically*. Rockville, MD: Aspen Systems.

Beckman, P. A. (1988, Spring). Budgeting for prepaid medicine. *College Review, 5*(1).

Feldman, S. (1992). *Managed mental health services*. Springfield, IL: Charles C Thomas.

Georgia Psychological Association. (1993, February). *Practical guide to billing and payment*. Atlanta, GA: Author.

How should your office look? (1992, August). *Interchange for Mental Health Professionals*, p. 4.

Love, J. D. (1992). Identifying applications for your office: Contracting for outside computer services. *Computers in Practice*, 36–37.

O'Connor, P. J., & M. A. Thomas Doyle. (1991). Corporate formula for health care. *Group Practice Journal.*

Psychotherapy Finances Staff. (1992). *Guide to private practice.* Jupiter, FL: Ridgewood Financial Institute, Inc.

Reinertsen, J. L. (1991). Transforming a group practice. *Group Practice Journal.*

Stoloff, M. L., Brewster, J., & Couch, J. V. (1991). *Hardware, software, and the mental health professional: The complete guide to office computerization.* Washington, DC: American Psychological Association.

Stoloff, M. L., & Couch, J. V. (1992). *Computer use in psychology: A directory of software* (3rd ed.). Washington, DC: American Psychological Association.

U.S. Department of Health and Human Services, Public Health Service, Alcohol, Drug Abuse, and Mental Health Administration. *Guidelines for the development and assessment of a comprehensive federal employee assistance program* (DHHS Publication No. ADM 88-1595). Washington, DC: U.S. Government Printing Office.

Glossary

ACCESS   An individual's ability to obtain medical or other human service agency services on a timely and financially acceptable basis.

ACUTE CARE   Inpatient, general routine care provided by hospitals or other facilities to patients who are ill but do not require the concentrated and continuous observation and care provided in the intensive care units of such institutions.

ADMINISTRATIVE SERVICES ONLY (ASO)   An arrangement under which an insurance carrier or an independent organization will, for a fee, handle the claims and benefits paperwork for a self-insured group (also see third-party administrator). In some states, the organizations supplying ASO can insure against a certain level of large, unpredictable claims (also see stop-loss).

ADVERSE SELECTION   Tendency for higher risk individuals to purchase health care and more comprehensive plans, resulting in increased costs; disproportionate insurance of risks who are poorer or more prone to suffer loss or make claims than the average risk.

AMBULATORY CARE   All types of health services that are provided on an outpatient basis. The term *ambulatory care* usually implies that the patient has come to a location to receive medical services and has departed the same day.

ANCILLARY SERVICES   Inpatient hospital services other than bed, board, and nursing care (e.g., drugs, dressings, operating room services, special diets, X-rays, laboratory examination, anesthesia, medications, etc.).

ASSIGNMENT   An agreement in which a patient assigns to another party, usually a provider or hospital, the right to receive payment from a public or private insurance program for the service that the patient has received. In Medicare, if a provider accepts assignment form the patient, he or she must agree to accept the program as payment in full (except for specific co-insurance, co-payment, and deductible amounts required of the patient).

AVERAGE LENGTH OF STAY (ALOS)   Number of days a patient customarily remains an inpatient for a specified diagnosis or procedure; used in precertification and recertification procedures.

BASIC HEALTH INSURANCE COVERAGE   Hospital and surgical–medical coverage; excludes major medical and dental coverage.

BASIC MEDICAL INSURANCE COVERAGE   First dollar provider coverage not subject to deductible or co-payment. It is usually based on usual and customary charges or an indemnity schedule.

BILL AUDITS   Some employers urge their employees to carefully examine all bills received (particularly from hospitals) to verify that all charges were for services rendered or supplies used. An incentive may be given; usually the employee receives a percentage of the money regained if an error is found.

CAPITATION   A method of payment for health care services in which the provider accepts a fixed amount of payment per subscriber, per period of time, in return for providing specified services over a specified period of time.

CARRIER Any commercial insurance company.

CARVE-OUT A program separate from the main group health plan designed to provide a specialized type of care, such as a mental health carve-out.

CASE MANAGEMENT A broad range of functions whereby covered individuals with specific health care needs are identified and a plan that efficiently utilizes health care resources is formulated and implemented to achieve the optimum client outcome in the most cost-effective manner.

CASE MANAGER A generic term for various professionals who perform different case management functions, usually working with clients, families, providers, and insurers to coordinate all services deemed necessary to provide the client with a plan of medically necessary and appropriate health care.

CHAMPUS Civilian Health and Medical Program of the Uniformed Services. A health plan of vast size with beneficiaries in all states and a natural field experiment in the use of mental health fee-for-services practices. The patterns of use have major public policy implications for consumers' access, providers' availability, the cost of alternatives to hospitalization, extent of use, and quality of care.

CHRONIC CARE Care provided to patients who have a continual or recurring illness, usually lengthy.

CLAIMS REVIEW A review of claims by government, medical foundations, professional review organizations, insurers, or others responsible for payment to determine liability and amount of payment.

CLOSED PANEL Medical services are delivered in the managed care organization (MCO)-owned health center or satellite clinic only by providers who belong to a specially formed but legally separate medical group that serves the MCO. The term usually refers to group and staff health maintenance organization models.

CO-INSURANCE The portion of charges the insured is responsible for, either the cost of covered services or of the monthly premium.

CONCURRENT PEER REVIEW (OR CONCURRENT UTILIZATION REVIEW) Monitoring of a provider's treatment and continued hospitalization of a patient performed by medical peers. Each hospital patient is given an initial length of stay (LOS) designation using locally determined criteria that are based on age, sex, and diagnosis. If a provider wishes to keep the patient beyond the designated LOS, it must be approved by those conducting the review. If an additional LOS is not approved, the patient may choose to continue hospitalization beyond the approved limit by assuming financial responsibility for the additional days of care.

CO-PAYMENT A type of cost sharing whereby insured or covered individuals pay a specified flat amount per unit of service or unit of time (e.g., $10 per visit, $25 per inpatient hospital day); insurance covers the remainder of the cost.

COST CONTAINMENT Actions taken by employers and insurers to curtail health care costs (e.g., increasing employee cost sharing, requiring second opinions, or preadmission screening).

COST SHARING   Requirement that health care consumers contribute to their own medical care costs through deductibles and co-insurance or co-payments.

COVERED EXPENSE (OR COVERED BENEFIT)   Health care costs that are specifically cited as reimbursable by the health plan.

CREDENTIALING   The process of reviewing a practitioner's credentials (i.e., training, experience, or demonstrated ability) for the purpose of determining whether criteria for clinical privileging are met.

DAYS/1,000/YEAR   This is a common utilization measurement used in the health care industry that refers to a ratio of the number of days a patient population has for a particular service per 1,000 members enrolled for a given year. For example, if a health maintenance organization with 10,000 members experiences 3,800 total hospital days, the relevant ratio is 380 hospital days per 1,000 members per years.

DAY TREATMENT   Intensive care provided at a facility only during the day. Patients in day treatment do not reside at the facility but instead return home.

DEDUCTIBLE   Flat sum that must be paid by the patient or employee before an insurer assumes liability for all or part of the remaining cost of covered services. A deductible is most commonly used in major medical policies.

DIAGNOSTIC-RELATED GROUPS (DRGs)   A reimbursement method whereby hospitals receive a fixed fee per patient on the basis of the admitting diagnosis regardless of length of stay or amount of service received.

DISCHARGE PLANNING   Process of identifying, monitoring, counseling, and arranging follow-up care of hospitalized patients. Usually performed by the treatment team or provider in charge, the process ensures patients receive appropriate counseling and follow-up care to assist their convalescence and keep hospital stays at a minimum.

EMPLOYEE ASSISTANCE PROGRAM (EAP)   An employer's program of counseling and other forms of assistance to employees experiencing alcoholism, substance abuse, or emotional and family problems.

ENROLLMENT   The means by which a person establishes membership in a group insurance plan.

EXCESS CHARGES   The portion of any charge greater than the usual and prevailing charge for a service. A charge is "usual and prevailing" when it does not exceed the typical charge of the provider in the absence of insurance and is no greater than the general level of charges for comparable services and supplies made by other providers in the same area.

EXCLUSIONS AND LIMITATIONS   Health and medical expenses that are specifically listed as not eligible for payment; often those costs might be covered under another insurance program such as worker's compensation or veterans benefits, personal in nature, or caused by military service.

EXCLUSIVE PROVIDER ORGANIZATION (EPO)   EPOs are similar to preferred provider organizations in their organization and purpose. However, beneficiaries covered by an EPO are required to receive all of their covered services from providers that participate in the EPO. The EPO does not cover services received from other providers. Some EPOs parallel health maintenance organizations in that they not only require exclusive use of the EPO provider network but also use a "gatekeeper" approach to authorize nonprimary care services.

EXPLANATION OF BENEFITS (EOB)   A form provided to patients (and providers) after a claim has been paid; useful in enabling the patient to check not only benefits received but also the services for which the provider has requested compensation. In Medicare, it is called "explanation of medical benefits" (EOMB).

FEE FOR SERVICE   Method of charging whereby a provider or other practitioner bills for each encounter or service rendered. This is the usual method of billing by the majority of providers. Under a fee-for-service payment system, expenditures increase not only if the fees themselves increase but also if more units of service are charged for or more expensive services are substituted for less expensive ones. The system contrasts with salary, per capita, or prepayment systems in which the payment is not changed with the number of services actually used or if none is used.

FREE-STANDING FACILITY   A health care center that is physically separated from a hospital or other institution of which it is a legal part or with which it is affiliated, or an independently operated or owned private or public business or enterprise providing a limited health care service or range such as ambulatory surgery, hemodialysis treatment, diagnostic tests or examinations, and so forth.

GATEKEEPING   The process by which a primary care provider directly provides the primary patient care and coordinates all diagnostic testing and specialty referrals required for a patient's medical care. Referrals must be preauthorized by the "gatekeeper" unless there is an emergency. Gatekeeping is a subset of the functions of the primary provider case manager.

GROUP CONTRACT   An arrangement between the managed care company and subscribing group containing rates, performance covenants, relationships among parties, schedule of benefits, and other conditions. The term is generally limited to a 12-month period but may be renewed.

GROUP HEALTH INSURANCE   A single program insuring a group of associated individuals against financial loss resulting from illness or injury.

GROUP MODEL   A health maintenance organization (HMO) model in which the HMO contracts with one or more provider groups on a capitation basis for the provision of services. The providers practice in a common facility and share staff. Income is pooled and distributed according to an agreed-on plan.

GROUP PRACTICE   A formal association of three or more health care providers providing services with income pooled and redistributed to members of the group through a prearranged plan.

HCFA Health Care Financing Administration. The federal agency within the U.S. Department of Health and Human Services responsible for administering the Medicare program.

HEALTH MAINTENANCE ORGANIZATION (HMO)   An entity that finances and furnishes designated health services needed by plan members for a fixed, prepaid premium. Services usually include primary care, emergency care, acute hospital care, extended care, and rehabilitation. There are four basic models of HMOs: group model, individual practice association, network model, and staff model. Under the federal HMO Act, an entity must have three characteristics: (a) an organized system of providing health care or otherwise ensuring health care delivery in a geographic area; (b) an agreed-on set of basic and supplemental health maintenance and treatment services; and (c) a voluntarily enrolled group of people.

HOLD HARMLESS CLAUSE   A clause frequently found in managed care contracts whereby the managed care organization and the provider hold each other not liable for malpractice or corporate malfeasance if either of the parties is found to be liable. Many insurance carriers exclude this type of liability from coverage. It may also refer to language that prohibits the provider from billing patients if their managed care company becomes insolvent. State and federal regulations may require this language.

INDEMNIFY   To make good a loss.

INDEMNITY BENEFITS   A fixed dollar payment for a specific health care service.

IDEPENDENT OR INDIVIDUAL PRACTICE ASSOCIATION (IPA)   A partnership, corporation, or association that has entered into an arrangement for provision of their services with individuals who are licensed to practice; one form of a health maintenance organization.

INTEGRATED CARE   An alternative delivery system developed by the American Psychological Association as a response to the rising costs of providing health care services. Based on six concepts: benefit design, case management and utilization review, communications, direct contracting, network development, and outcomes.

MANAGED CARE   A means of providing health care services within a defined network of health care providers who are given the responsibility to manage and provide care. Increasingly, the term is being used by many analysts to include (in addition to health maintenance organizations) preferred provider organizations and even forms of indemnity insurance coverage that incorporate preadmission certifications and other utilization controls.

MANAGED COMPETITION   A health care reform proposal that would restructure the present market so that small purchasers would have the same purchasing power as larger groups. The market would be "regulated" via competition between accountable health plans attempting to serve large health insurance purchasing cooperatives, which would represent a large percentage of the insured population for a given location.

MANDATED BENEFITS   Specific treatments, providers, or individuals required by law to be included in commercial health plans.

MARKET SHARE   That part of the market potential that a managed care company has captured; usually market share is expressed as a percentage of the market potential.

MEDICAID   The federally financed, state-run health care program for economically disadvantaged individuals.

MEDICARE   Title XVIII of the Social Security Act, which provides benefits to citizens aged 65 and older and to disabled individuals. Part A covers hospitalization, extended care, and nursing home care. Part B provides medical–surgical benefits.

MENTAL HEALTH AND DRUG ABUSE SERVICES   There are three basic types of mental health services: inpatient care provided in short-term psychiatric beds in a general hospital or in specialized psychiatric facilities, outpatient care for individual or group counseling, partial hospitalization, or a combination of all three. Also see employee assistance programs.

MULTISPECIALTY GROUP   A group of practitioners who represent various specialties and who work together in a group practice.

NETWORK MODEL   An organizational form in which the health maintenance organization (HMO) contracts for medical services within a "network" of medical groups. HealthNet, a Blue Cross-sponsored HMO serving southern California, is an example of a network model. For federal qualification purposes, such models are designated as individual practice associations.

OUT OF AREA BENEFITS   The coverage allowed to health maintenance organization (HMO) members for emergency situations outside of the prescribed geographic area of the HMO.

OUT OF AREA CARE   Care received by a health maintenance organization's (HMO's) enrollees when they are outside the HMO's geographic territory. Services received are usually not prearranged by the HMO.

PEER REVIEW   Ideally, evaluation by practicing providers (or other qualified professionals) of the quality and efficiency of services ordered or performed by other practicing providers. *Peer review* is the all-inclusive term for medical review efforts. Medical practice, inpatient hospital and extended care facility analyses, utilization review, medical audit, ambulatory care, and claims review are all aspects of peer review.

PERFORMANCE STANDARDS   Standards an individual provider is expected to meet, especially with respect to quality of care. The standards may define volume of care delivered per time period.

POINT-OF-SERVICE PLAN (POS)   A combination of some features of a health maintenance organization (HMO) and a preferred provider organization. Although there are other variations, in most cases members elect a primary care provider who manages a patient's care. However, members have the option to seek care from outside the POS network at a lower reimbursement level. Most HMOs are introducing POS products as a means of attracting greater market share than they can with the traditional "lock in" product.

POOL   A large number of small groups or individuals that are analyzed and rated as a single large group for insurance purposes. A risk pool may be any account that attempts to find the claims liability for a group with a common denominator.

PREADMISSION REVIEW   When a provider requests that a patient be hospitalized, another opinion may be sought. The second provider reviews the treatment plan and evaluates the patient's condition and confirms the request for admission or recommends another course of action. Similar to second opinions on surgery.

PREAUTHORIZATION   Review and approval of covered benefits done on the basis of a provider's treatment plan. Some insurers require preauthorization for certain high-cost procedures. Other insurers apply the preauthorization requirement when charges are in excess of a specified dollar amount.

PRECERTIFICATION   A review of the necessity and length of a recommended hospital stay. Certification prior to admission is often required for all nonemergencies and certification within 48 hours following admission for emergency treatment.

PREEXISTING CONDITION   Any condition for which charges have been incurred during a specified period of time just prior to the effective date of an insurance policy. Frequently, a contract with a different insurer will not cover the preexisting conditions of employees or their dependents.

PREFERRED PROVIDER ORGANIZATION (PPO)   PPOs are entities through which employer health benefit plans and health insurance carriers contract to purchase health care services for covered beneficiaries from a selected group of preferred providers. Usually, the benefit contract provides significantly better benefits for services received from preferred providers, thus encouraging members to use these providers. Members are also generally allowed benefits for nonparticipating providers' services, usually on an indemnity basis with significant co-payments. A PPO arrangement can be insured or self-funded. Providers may be, but are not necessarily, paid on a discounted fee-for-service basis.

PROFESSIONAL REVIEW ORGANIZATION (PRO)   An organized group of providers with the responsibility of reviewing and evaluating the ethics and quality of services rendered by the provider community within a defined geographic area. An organization in which practicing providers assume responsibility for reviewing the propriety and quality of health care services provided under Medicare and Medicaid.

QUALITY ASSURANCE   Activities and programs intended to ensure the quality of care in a defined medical setting or program. Such programs include methods for documenting clinical practice, educational components intended to remedy identified deficiencies in quality, as well as the components necessary to identify and correct such deficiencies (e.g., peer or utilization review) and formal processes to assess the program's own effectiveness.

QUALITY MANAGEMENT   An intervention in which all employees and managers continuously review the quality of the service they provide. The process used identifies problems, tests solutions to those problems, and constantly monitors the solutions for improvement.

RATING   The process of determining rates or the cost of insurance for individuals, groups, or classes of risks.

RESIDENTIAL CARE   Care provided in a residential treatment center or group home 24 hours a day.

RISK   The chance or possibility of loss. The sharing of risk is often employed as a utilization control mechanism within the health maintenance organization setting. Risk is often defined in insurance terms as the possibility of loss associated with a given population.

RISK POOL   A pool of money that is to be used for defined expenses. Commonly, if the money that is put at risk is not expended by the end of the year, some or all of it is returned to those managing the risk.

SELF-FUNDING   A procedure whereby a firm uses its own funds to pay claims rather than transferring the financial risks of paying claims to an outside insurer in exchange for premium payment. Also referred to as self-insurance. Insurance companies and other third-party administrator organizations may be engaged to process claims, or the self-insured company may choose to handle its own. Four forms of claims administration are common:

COST PLUS   Third party pays claims and bills the employer for the actual amount of claims in a month (cost) plus an administrative fee to a carrier (plus).

ADMINISTRATIVE SERVICES ONLY (ASO)   Employer contracts with a firm to handle claims and make payments for billed services.

SELF-ADMINISTRATION   Employer takes on the risk for claims and does the administrative work involved in paying claims.

MINIMUM PREMIUM PLAN   Insurance company provides aggregate stop-loss protection plus claims administration services.

STAFF MODEL   In this organizational model, the health plan employs providers who provide or arrange for the provision of covered services to health plan enrollees. In certain instances, this type of health plan will subcontract with an individual practitioner or practitioner group to provide services that employed providers cannot provide or are unavailable to provide.

STOP-LOSS COVERAGE   Insurance for a self-insured plan that reimburses the company for any losses it might incur in its health claims beyond a specified amount.

THIRD-PARTY PAYOR   Any organization, public or private, that pays or insures health or medical expenses on behalf of beneficiaries or recipients. The individual generally pays a premium for such coverage in all private and some public programs. The organization then pays the bills on the individual's behalf; such payments are called third-party payments and are distinguished by the separation between the individual receiving the services (the first party) and the organization paying for it (the third party).

THIRD-PARTY ADMINISTRATOR (TPA)   Outside company responsible for handling claims and performing administrative tasks associated with health insurance plan maintenance.

USUAL, CUSTOMARY, AND REASONABLE (UCR)   Health insurance plans that pay a provider's full charge if it is reasonable and does not exceed his or her usual charges and the amount customarily charged for service by other providers in the area.

UTILIZATION REVIEW (UR)   A review of records of patients on a sampling or other basis to determine conformity with reasonable standards for use of health resources; involves length-of-stay review as well as appropriateness of hospital admissions and misuse and overuse of services. UR may be performed prior to hospitalization (preadmission review), during a hospital stay (concurrent review), or prospectively (quality review, evaluation studies). Reviews may be initiated by insurance carriers, alternate delivery system organizations, employers, or third-party administrators and are usually conducted by groups of providers, often organized by provider societies or private consulting firms and universities.